# Surgery: Complications, Risks and Consequences

*Series Editor*
Brendon J. Coventry

For further volumes:
http://www.springer.com/series/11761

Brendon J. Coventry
Editor

# Pediatric Surgery

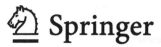 Springer

*Editor*
Brendon J. Coventry, BMBS, PhD,
FRACS, FACS, FRSM
Discipline of Surgery
Royal Adelaide Hospital
University of Adelaide
Adelaide, SA
Australia

ISBN 978-1-4471-7086-0      ISBN 978-1-4471-5439-6   (eBook)
DOI 10.1007/978-1-4471-5439-6
Springer London Heidelberg New York Dordrecht

*This book is dedicated to my wonderful wife Christine and children Charles, Cameron, Alexander and Eloise who make me so proud, having supported me through this mammoth project; my patients, past, present and future; my numerous mentors, teachers, colleagues, friends and students, who know who they are; my parents Beryl and Lawrence; and my parents-in-law Barbara and George, all of whom have taught me and encouraged me to achieve*

*"Without love and understanding we have but nothing"*

*Brendon J. Coventry*

# Foreword I

This comprehensive treatise is remarkable for its breadth and scope and its authorship by global experts. Indeed, knowledge of its content is essential if we are to achieve optimal and safe outcomes for our patients. The content embodies the details of our surgical discipline and how to incorporate facts and evidence into our surgical judgment as well as recommendations to our patients.

While acknowledging that the technical aspects of surgery are its distinguishing framework of our profession, the art and judgment of surgery requires an in depth knowledge of biology, anatomy, pathophysiology, clinical science, surgical outcomes and complications that distinguishes the theme of this book. This knowledge is essential to assure us that we are we doing the right operation, at the right time, and in the right patient. In turn, that knowledge is essential to take into account how surgical treatment interfaces with the correct sequence and combination with other treatment modalities. It is also essential to assess the extent of scientific evidence from clinical trials and surgical expertise that is the underpinning of our final treatment recommendation to our patient.

Each time I sit across from a patient to make a recommendation for a surgical treatment, I am basing my recommendation on a "benefit/risk ratio" that integrates scientific evidence, and my intuition gained through experience. That is, do the potential benefits outweigh the potential risks and complications as applied to an individual patient setting? The elements of that benefit/ risk ratio that are taken into account include: the natural history of the disease, the stage/extent of disease, scientific and empirical evidence of treatment outcomes, quality of life issues (as perceived by the patient), co-morbidity that might influence surgical outcome, risks and complications inherent to the operation (errors of commission) and the risk(s) of not proceeding with an operation (errors of omission).

Thus, if we truly want to improve our surgical outcomes, then we must understand and be able to either avoid, or execute sound management of, any complications that occur (regardless of whether they are due to co-morbidity or iatrogenic causes), to get our patent safely through the operation and its post-operative course. These subjects are nicely incorporated into the content of this book.

I highly recommend this book as a practical yet comprehensive treatise for the practicing surgeon and the surgical trainee. It is well organized, written with great clarity and nicely referenced when circumstances require further information.

Charles M. Balch, MD, FACS
Professor of Surgery
University of Texas, Southwestern Medical Center,
Dallas, TX, USA
Formerly, Professor of Surgery, Johns Hopkins Hospital,
Baltimore, MD, USA
Formerly, Executive Vice President and CEO,
American Society of Clinical Oncology (ASCO)
Past-President, Society of Surgical Oncology (USA)

# Foreword II

Throughout my clinical academic career I have aspired to improve the quality and safety of my surgical and clinical practice. It is very clear, while reading this impressive collection and synthesis of high-impact clinical evidence and international expert consensus, that in this new textbook, Brendon Coventry has the ambition to innovate and advance the quality and safety of surgical discipline.

In these modern times, where we find an abundance of information that is available through the internet, and of often doubtful authenticity, it is vital that we retain a professional responsibility for the collection, analysis and dissemination of evidenced-based and accurate knowledge and guidance to benefit both clinicians and our patients.

This practical and broad-scoped compendium, which contains over 250 procedures and their related complications and associated risks, will undoubtedly become a benchmark to raise the safety and quality of surgical practice for all that read it. It also manages to succeed in providing a portal for all surgeons, at any stage of their careers, to reflect on the authors' own combined experiences and the collective insights of a strong and influential network of peers.

This text emphasizes the need to understand and appreciate our patients and the intimate relationship that their physiology, co-morbidities and underlying diagnosis can have upon their unique surgical risk with special regard to complications and adverse events.

I recognize that universally across clinical practice and our profession, the evidence base and guidance to justify our decision-making is growing, but there is also a widening gap between what we know and what we do. The variation that we see in the quality of practice throughout the world should not be tolerated.

This text makes an assertive contribution to promote quality by outlining the prerequisite foundational knowledge of surgery, science and anatomy and their complex interactions with clinical outcome that is needed for all in the field of surgery.

I thoroughly recommend this expertly constructed collection. Its breadth and quality is a testament to its authors and editor.

Professor the Lord Ara Darzi, PC, KBE, FRCS, FRS
Paul Hamlyn Chair of Surgery
Imperial College London, London, UK
Formerly Undersecretary of State for Health,
Her Majesty's Government, UK

# Conditions of Use and Disclaimer

Information is provided *for improved medical education and potential improvement in clinical practice only*. The information is based on composite material from research studies and professional personal opinion and does not guarantee accuracy for any specific clinical situation or procedure. There is also *no express or implied guarantee to accuracy or that surgical complications will be prevented, minimized, or reduced* in any way. The advice is *intended for use by individuals with suitable professional qualifications* and education in medical practice and the ability to apply the knowledge in a suitable manner for a specific condition or disease, and in an appropriate clinical context. The data is complex by nature and open to some interpretation. The purpose is to assist medical practitioners to improve awareness of possible complications, risks or consequences associated with surgical procedures for the benefit of those practitioners in the improved care of their patients. The application of the information contained herein for a specific patient or problem must be performed with care to ensure that the situation and advice is appropriate and correct for that patient and situation. The material is expressly *not for medico-legal purposes*.

The information contained in *Surgery: Complications, Risks and Consequences* is provided for the purpose of improving consent processes in healthcare and in no way guarantees prevention, early detection, risk reduction, economic benefit or improved practice of surgical treatment of any disease or condition.

The information provided in *Surgery: Complications, Risks and Consequences* is of a general nature and is not a substitute for independent medical advice or research in the management of particular diseases or patient situations by health care professionals. It should not be taken as replacing or overriding medical advice.

The Publisher or *Copyright* holder does not accept any liability for any injury, loss, delay or damage incurred arising from use, misuse, interpretation, omissions or reliance on the information provided in *Surgery: Complications, Risks and Consequences* directly or indirectly.

## Currency and Accuracy of Information

The user should always check that any information acted upon is up-to-date and accurate. Information is provided in good faith and is **subject to change and alter-ation without notice**. Every effort is made with *Surgery: Complications, Risks and Consequences* to provide current information, but no warranty, guarantee or legal responsibility is given that information provided or referred to has not changed without the knowledge of the publisher, editor or authors. Always check the quality of information provided or referred to for accuracy for the situation where it is intended to be used, or applied. We do, however, attempt to provide useful and valid information. Because of the broad nature of the information provided incomplete-ness or omissions of specific or general complications may have occured and users must take this into account when using the text. No responsibility is taken for delayed, missed or inaccurate diagnosis of any illness, disease or health state at any time.

## External Web Site Links or References

The decisions about the accuracy, currency, reliability and correctness of informa-tion made by individuals using the *Surgery: Complications, Risks and Consequences* information or from external Internet links remain the individuals own concern and responsibility. Such external links or reference materials or other information should not be taken as an endorsement, agreement or recommendation of any third party products, services, material, information, views or content offered by these sites or publications. Users should check the sources and validity of information obtained for themselves prior to use.

## Privacy and Confidentiality

We maintain confidentiality and privacy of personal information but do not guaran-tee any confidentiality or privacy.

## Errors or Suggested Changes

If you or any colleagues note any errors or wish to suggest changes please notify us directly as they would be gratefully received.

# How to Use This Book

This book provides a resource for better understanding of surgical procedures and potential complications in general terms. The application of this material will depend on the individual patient and clinical context. It is not intended to be absolutely comprehensive for all situations or for all patients, but act as a 'guide' for understanding and prediction of complications, to assist in risk management and improvement of patient outcomes.

The design of the book is aimed at:

- Reducing Risk and better Managing Risks associated with surgery
- Providing information about 'general complications' associated with surgery
- Providing information about 'specific complications' associated with surgery
- Providing comprehensive information in one location, to assist surgeons in their explanation to the patient during the consent process

For each specific surgical procedure the text provides:

- Description and some background of the surgical procedure
- Anatomical points and possible variations
- Estimated Frequencies
- Perspective
- Major Complications

From this, a better understanding of the risks, complications and consequences associated with surgical procedures can hopefully be gained by the clinician for explanation of relevant and appropriate aspects to the patient.

The *Estimated frequency lists are not mean't to be totally comprehensive* or to contain all of the information that needs to be explained in obtaining informed consent from the patient for a surgical procedure. Indeed, *most of the information is for the surgeon* or reader only, *not designed for the patient*, however, parts should be selected by the surgeon at their discretion for appropriate explanation to the individual patient in the consent process.

Many patients would not understand or would be confused by the number of potential complications that may be associated with a specific surgical procedure, so ***some degree of selective discussion of the risks, complications and consequences would be necessary and advisable,*** as would usually occur in clinical practice. This judgement should necessarily be left to the surgeon, surgeon-in-training or other practitioner.

# Preface

Over the last decade or so we have witnessed a rapid change in the consumer demand for information by patients preparing for a surgical procedure. This is fuelled by multiple factors including the 'internet revolution', altered public consumer attitudes, professional patient advocacy, freedom of information laws, insurance issues, risk management, and medicolegal claims made through the legal system throughout the western world, so that the need has arisen for a higher, fairer and clearer standard of *'informed consent'*.

One of the my main difficulties encountered as a young intern, and later as a surgical resident, registrar and consultant surgeon, was obtaining information for use for the pre-operative consenting of patients, and for managing patients on the ward after surgical operations. I watched others struggle with the same problem too. The literature contained many useful facts and clinical studies, but it was unwieldy and very time-consuming to access, and the information that was obtained seemed specific to well-defined studies of highly specific groups of patients. These patient studies, while useful, often did not address my particular patient under treatment in the clinic, operating theatre or ward. Often the studies came from centres with vast experience of a particular condition treated with one type of surgical procedure, constituting a series or trial.

What I wanted to know was:

- The **main complications** associated with a surgical procedure;
- **Information that could be provided** during the consent process, and
- How to **reduce the relative risks** of a complication, where possible

This information was difficult to find in one place!

As a young surgeon, on a very long flight from Adelaide to London, with much time to think and fuelled by some very pleasant champagne, I started making some notes about how I might tackle this problem. My first draft was idle scribble, as I listed the ways surgical complications could be classified. After finding over 10 different classification systems for listing complications, the task became much larger and more complex. I then realized why someone had not taken on this job before!

After a brief in-flight sleep and another glass, the task became far less daunting and suddenly much clearer – the champagne was very good, and there was little else to do in any case!

It was then that I decided to speak with as many of my respected colleagues as I could from around the globe, to get their opinions and advice. The perspectives that emerged were remarkable, as many of them had faced the same dilemmas in their own practices and hospitals, also without a satisfactory solution.

What developed was a composite documentation of information (i) from the published literature and (ii) from the opinions of many experienced surgical practitioners in the field – to provide a text to supply information on **Complications, Risks and Consequences of Surgery** for surgical and other clinical practitioners to use at the bedside and in the clinic.

This work represents the culmination of more than 10 years work with the support and help of colleagues from around the world, for the benefit of their students, junior surgical colleagues, peers, and patients. To them, I owe much gratitude for their cooperation, advice, intellect, experience, wise counsel, friendship and help, for their time, and for their continued encouragement in this rather long-term and complex project. I have already used the text material myself with good effect and it has helped me enormously in my surgical practice.

The text aims to provide health professionals with useful information, which can be selectively used to better inform patients of the potential surgical complications, risks and consequences. I sincerely hope it fulfils this role.

Adelaide, SA, Australia                                    Brendon J. Coventry, BMBS, PhD,
                                                                              FRACS, FACS, FRSM

# Acknowledgments

I wish to thank:

The many learned friends and experienced colleagues who have contributed in innumerable ways along the way in the writing of this text.

Professor Sir Peter Morris, formerly Professor of Surgery at Oxford University, and also Past-President of the College of Surgeons of England, for allowing me to base my initial work at the Nuffield Department of Surgery (NDS) and John Radcliffe Hospital in the University of Oxford, for the UK sector of the studies. He and his colleagues have provided encouragement and valuable discussion time over the course of the project.

The (late) Professor John Farndon, Professor of Surgery at the University of Bristol, Bristol Royal Infirmary, UK; and Professor Robert Mansel, Professor of Surgery at the University of Wales, Cardiff, UK for discussions and valued advice.

Professor Charles Balch, then Professor of Surgery at the Johns Hopkins University, Baltimore, Maryland, USA, and Professor Clifford Ko, from UCLA and American College of Surgeons NSQIP Program, USA, for helpful discussions.

Professor Armando Guiliano, formerly of the John Wayne Cancer Institute, Santa Monica, California, USA for his contributions and valuable discussions.

Professor Jonathan Meakins, then Professor of Surgery at McGill University, Quebec, Canada, who provided helpful discussions and encouragement, during our respective sabbatical periods, which coincided in Oxford; and later as Professor of Surgery at Oxford University.

Over the last decade, numerous clinicians have discussed and generously contributed their experience to the validation of the range and relative frequency of complications associated with the wide spectrum of surgical procedures. These clinicians include:

*Los Angeles, USA*: Professor Carmack Holmes, Cardiothoracic Surgeon, Los Angeles (UCLA); Professor Donald Morton, Melanoma Surgeon, Los Angeles; Dr R Essner, Melanoma Surgeon, Los Angeles.

*New York, USA*: Professor Murray Brennan; Dr David Jacques; Prof L Blumgart; Dr Dan Coit; Dr Mary Sue Brady (Surgeons, Department of Surgery, Memorial Sloan-Kettering Cancer Centre, New York);

*Oxford, UK*: Dr Linda Hands, Vascular Surgeon; Dr Jack Collin, Vascular Surgeon; Professor Peter Friend, Transplant and Vascular Surgeon; Dr Nick Maynard, Upper Gastrointestinal Surgeon; Dr Mike Greenall, Breast Surgeon; Dr Jane Clark, Breast Surgeon; Professor Derek Gray, Vascular/Pancreatic Surgeon; Dr Julian Britton, Hepato-Biliary Surgeon; Dr Greg Sadler, Endocrine Surgeon; Dr Christopher Cunningham, Colorectal Surgeon; Professor Neil Mortensen, Colorectal Surgeon; Dr Bruce George, Colorectal Surgeon; Dr Chris Glynn, Anaesthetist (National Health Service (NHS), Oxford, UK).

*Bristol, UK*: Professor Derek Alderson.

*Adelaide, Australia*: Professor Guy Ludbrook, Anesthetist; Dr Elizabeth Tam, Anesthetist.

A number of senior medical students at the University of Adelaide, including Hwee Sim Tan, Adelaine S Lam, Ramon Pathi, Mohd Azizan Ghzali, William Cheng, Sue Min Ooi, Teena Silakong, and Balaji Rajacopalin, who assisted during their student projects in the preliminary feasibility studies and research, and their participation is much appreciated. Thanks also to numerous sixth year students, residents and surgeons at Hospitals in Adelaide who participated in questionnaires and surveys.

The support of the University of Adelaide, especially the Department of Surgery, and Royal Adelaide Hospital has been invaluable in allowing the sabbatical time to engineer the collaborations necessary for this project to progress. I thank Professors Glyn Jamieson and Guy Maddern for their support in this regard.

I especially thank the Royal Australasian College of Surgeons for part-support through the Marjorie Hooper Fellowship.

I thank my clinical colleagues on the Breast, Endocrine and Surgical Oncology Unit at the Royal Adelaide Hospital, especially Grantley Gill, James Kollias and Melissa Bochner, for caring for my patients and assuming greater clinical load when I have been away.

Professor Bill Runciman, Australian Patient Safety Foundation, for all of his advice and support; Professors Cliff Hughes and Bruce Barraclough, from the Royal Australasian College of Surgeons, the Clinical Excellence Commission, New South Wales, and the Australian Commission (Council) on Safety and Quality in Healthcare.

Thanks too to Kai Holt, Anne-Marie Bennett and Carrie Cooper who assisted and helped to organise my work. I also acknowledge my collaborator Martin Ashdown for being so patient during distractions from our scientific research work. Also to Graeme Cogdell, Imagart Design Ltd, Adelaide, for his expertise and helpful discussions.

I particularly thank Melissa Morton and her global team at Springer-Verlag for their work in preparing the manuscript for publication.

Importantly, I truly appreciate and thank my wife Christine, my four children and our parents/ wider family for their support in every way towards seeing this project through to its completion, and in believing so much in me, and in my work.

Adelaide, SA, Australia                                      Brendon J. Coventry, BMBS, PhD,
                                                                              FRACS, FACS, FRSM

# Contents

# Contributors

**Jayme Bennetts, BMBS, FRACS, FCSANZ** Cardiac and Thoracic Surgery, Flinders Medical Centre, Adelaide, Australia

**Hilary Boucaut, MBBS, FRACS** Urology Unit, Women's and Children's Hospital, Adelaide, Australia

**Brendon J. Coventry, BMBS, PhD, FRACS, FACS, FRSM** Discipline of Surgery, Royal Adelaide Hospital, University of Adelaide, Adelaide, SA, Australia

**Andrew Davidson, MBBS, FANZCA, GradDipEdBiostat, MD** Royal Children's Hospital, The University of Melbourne, Melbourne, Australia

**Andrew Ford, MB, ChB, ChM, FRCSEd, FRCS, FRACS** Division of Paediatric Surgery (Chief of Surgery), Women's and Children's Hospital, Adelaide, Australia

**John Hutson, BS, MD, FRACS, DSc, FRAP (hon)** Department of Paediatrics, Royal Children's Hospital, Melbourne, Australia

**Christopher Kirby, FRCS, FRACS** Department of Paediatric Surgery, Women's and Children's Hospital, Adelaide, Australia

**Catherine N. Olweny, BA(hon), BMBS, FANZCA** Department of Anaesthesia and Pain Management, The Royal Children's Hospital, Melbourne, Australia

**Christine Russell, BA, BM, BCh, FRACS** Central and Northern Adelaide Renal and Transplantation Service, Royal Adelaide Hospital, Adelaide, Australia

**Anthony L. Sparnon, MBBS, FRACS** Women's and Children's Hospital, North Adelaide, Australia

# Chapter 1
# Introduction

Brendon J. Coventry

This volume deals with complications, risks, and consequences related to a range of procedures under the broad headings of pediatric anesthesia, pediatric abdominal surgery, pediatric tumor surgery, pediatric thoracic surgery, pediatric vascular access surgery, and pediatric urological surgery.

**Important Note**

It should be emphasized that the risks and frequencies that are given here *represent derived figures*. These *figures are best estimates of relative frequencies across most institutions*, not merely the highest-performing ones, and as such are often representative of a number of studies, which include different patients with differing comorbidities and different surgeons. In addition, the risks of complications in lower- or higher-risk patients may lie outside these estimated ranges, and individual clinical judgment is required as to the expected risks communicated to the patient and staff or for other purposes. The range of risks is also derived from experience and the literature; while risks outside this range may exist, certain risks may be reduced or absent due to variations of procedures or surgical approaches. It is recognized that different patients, practitioners, institutions, regions, and countries may vary in their requirements and recommendations.

Individual clinical judgment should always be exercised, of course, when applying the general information contained in these documents to individual patients in a clinical setting.

B.J. Coventry, BMBS, PhD, FRACS, FACS, FRSM
Discipline of Surgery, Royal Adelaide Hospital, University of Adelaide,
L5 Eleanor Harrald Building, North Terrace, 5000 Adelaide, SA, Australia
e-mail: brendon.coventry@adelaide.edu.au

B.J. Coventry (ed.), *Pediatric Surgery*, Surgery: Complications, Risks and Consequences,    1
DOI 10.1007/978-1-4471-5439-6_1, © Springer-Verlag London 2014

# Chapter 2
# Pediatric Anesthesia for Surgery

**Catherine N. Olweny, Andrew Davidson, Christopher Kirby, John Hutson, and Brendon J. Coventry**

## Overview

Pediatric surgery is performed in preterm infants through to adult-size teenagers. In broad terms, pediatric surgery is performed almost exclusively under general anesthesia. The pediatric age range covers a multitude of rapid physiological changes that occur with growth, not the least of which are the "size" and "mental maturity" of the patient. Therefore, the type of anesthesia and approaches used will often vary with the type of surgery and with the age and size of the patient. The coexistence of other anomalies, some of which may themselves be life threatening, adds another layer of complexity to pediatric anesthesia and surgery. The chapter is not designed to be fully comprehensive in the discussion of anesthesia, but many of the important principles are considered.

C.N. Olweny, BA(hon), BMBS, FANZCA
Department of Anaesthesia and Pain Management, The Royal Children's Hospital, Melbourne, Australia

A. Davidson, MBBS, FANZCA, GradDipEdBiostat, MD
Royal Children's Hospital, The University of Melbourne, Melbourne, Australia

C. Kirby, FRCS, FRACS
Department of Paediatric Surgery, Women's and Children's Hospital, Adelaide, Australia

J. Hutson, BS, MD, FRACS, DSc, FRAP(hon)
Department of Paediatrics, Royal Children's Hospital, Melbourne, Australia

B.J. Coventry, BMBS, PhD, FRACS, FACS, FRSM (✉)
Discipline of Surgery, Royal Adelaide Hospital, University of Adelaide,
L5 Eleanor Harrald Building, North Terrace, 5000 Adelaide, SA, Australia
e-mail: brendon.coventry@adelaide.edu.au

B.J. Coventry (ed.), *Pediatric Surgery*, Surgery: Complications, Risks and Consequences,
DOI 10.1007/978-1-4471-5439-6_2, © Springer-Verlag London 2014

**Important Note**
It should be emphasized that the risks and frequencies that are given here *represent derived figures*. These *figures are best estimates of relative frequencies across most institutions*, not merely the highest-performing ones, and as such are often representative of a number of studies, which include different patients with differing comorbidities and different surgeons. In addition, the risks of complications in lower- or higher-risk patients may lie outside these estimated ranges, and individual clinical judgment is required as to the expected risks communicated to the patient and staff or for other purposes. The range of risks is also derived from experience and the literature; while risks outside this range may exist, certain risks may be reduced or absent due to variations of procedures or surgical approaches. It is recognized that different patients, practitioners, institutions, regions, and countries may vary in their requirements and recommendations.

# Introduction

Anatomical, physiological, and psychological differences create challenges that are unique to pediatric surgery and anesthesia. This chapter aims to discuss the anatomical and physiological factors that affect the conduct of anesthesia in pediatric patients and to relate the important psychological aspects of dealing with anesthesia and surgery in children. Specific issues that occur in the preoperative, intraoperative, and postoperative management of pediatric patients are reviewed.

# Psychological Aspects

Mental maturity among pediatric patients ranges from infants and preschool children to school-aged children and teenagers. In addition, pediatric care is unique in that it essentially involves caring for the family. The perioperative period is one of anxiety for both parents and children with induction of anesthesia likely to be the most stressful time (Chorney and Kain 2010). There should be a dedicated pediatric admission and preoperative area. Ideally there should be separate areas for infants and preschool children, school-aged children, and teenagers. There should also be a dedicated pediatric recovery and postoperative area. The staff in these areas should be trained and experienced in managing the specific needs of pediatric patients prior to anesthesia and surgery and during the recovery period.

## Consent Procedures

Many jurisdictions prescribe that children up to a given age are unable to legally give consent for most surgical procedures. This means that children under the prescribed legal age will require the consent of a parent, guardian, or legal caregiver before anesthesia or surgery can be performed. The age at which legal consent is permitted depends upon the particular jurisdiction where the informed consent for anesthesia or surgical procedure is being obtained and the reasons for seeking the consent. Special statutes often exist to provide consent for emergency life-threatening procedures where urgency is paramount or where the appropriate legal consent cannot be reasonably obtained in a timely manner. In many jurisdictions, the opinions and consent of two legally qualified medical practitioners are sufficient for emergency procedures to proceed, if parental consent remains unobtainable.

This situation surrounding legal consent for surgical procedures means that instead of one patient, there are effectively two or more interested parties all of whom require some form of explanation of the intended procedure. The child may require a simplified explanation, while the parent or guardian will require a detailed explanation to gain a suitable understanding to enable "informed," "third-party" consent to be given. The person accompanying the child into the hospital or doctor's surgery may not be the person charged with the legal power to give the consent. The legal adequacy of the person providing the consent for the child needs to be confirmed. This may cause some delays in provision of the consent. If appropriate, it is preferable to have a delay rather than a nonlegally binding consent for anesthesia or surgery, should any problems later arise. Telephone consent may be appropriate but may be fraught with problems related to verification of the identity of the person providing consent. In these situations, agreed confirmation by another senior member of the staff listening to the conversation may be appropriate. The surgeon and anesthetist can perform this task, or a separate medical/nursing party may be included.

In simple terms, the parent or guardian should:

(i) Be asked whether they have the legal guardianship of the child
(ii) Be informed what the intended procedure is
(iii) Be informed that other procedures may be required in the course of surgery and what these might include
(iv) Be informed what the consequences might be from not operating and of any other operative or nonoperative options that may be sensible in the situation
(v) Be informed what the complications, consequences, and risks of the intended procedure might include
(vi) Be informed what the likely postoperative course might entail (e.g., ICU, hospital length of stay, further surgery, drains, tubes, feeding)

# Anatomical Considerations

## Body Size

The size of the child determines the size of the body parts that are being operated upon and consequently may impose difficulty of access and demand delicacy in tissue handling. Gut tubes and organs are smaller, and the size of vessels and airways is likewise smaller. These facts increase the challenges of anastomotic formation and cannulation for vascular access.

## Surgical Incisions

Children have wider rather than longer abdominal dimensions than adults, and so it is common to use transverse incisions for abdominal access. This means that retraction is often in a superior direction from over the child's head, especially in neonates and the smaller child. The assistant may unintentionally apply pressure on the face, the endotracheal tube, intravenous sites, or the chest. This may dislodge tubes or even cause injury to the child. The chest of the small child is likewise wider rather than longer in its dimensions, and the rib cage is highly flexible because the bone has not yet formed to stiffen the chest wall. Care needs to be taken not to compress the chest wall during surgery as significant compression can result in impaired ventilation. This is particularly important during thoracotomy where retraction of the lung is utilized to gain surgical access. Lung isolation and collapse is not used due to the narrow airways and difficulties of double-lumen tubes.

## Thermoregulation

Under general and regional anesthesia, the thermoregulatory response to hypothermia is absent. Vasodilation leads to a redistribution of heat from the core to the periphery and heat loss occurs by conduction, convection, radiation, and evaporation. In infants, small children, and in particular preterm babies, the large surface area to body weight ratio and paucity of subcutaneous fat increase the rate of heat loss (Hillier et al. 2004). Surgical exposure can be large relative to the size of the patient further increasing heat loss. Without active warming and measures to reduce heat loss, hypothermia is inevitable under general anesthesia and ensues rapidly in pediatric patients. Hypothermia causes reduced enzyme function leading to prolonged action of drugs including muscle relaxants. Hypothermia also leads to coagulopathy, impaired platelet function, and increased nonsurgical bleeding. Hypothermia is associated with arrhythmias, increased metabolic demand (Hillier et al. 2004), and increased incidence of wound infection. Hypothermia can also lead to delayed awakening from anesthesia and prolonged stay in the postanesthesia care unit. It is imperative to minimize heat loss by raising the ambient temperature, by covering the patient where possible, and by using warmed irrigation fluids and intravenous fluids. Overhead radiant heating of neonates is commonplace in many pediatric operating theaters. Modern active warming methods such as forced air warmers are effective and can raise an infant's temperature rapidly. Monitoring body temperature is important in order to avoid both hypothermia and hyperthermia from active warming.

## Physiological Considerations

### *Respiratory*

The airway and respiratory system of neonates and infants have anatomical and functional differences that affect the conduct of anesthesia and surgery. Infants have a large head relative to body size, relatively large tongues, and narrow nasal passages. Positioning the pediatric patient for effective mask ventilation and intubation does not require a pillow. Bag mask ventilation requires an open mouth and a delicate hand avoiding submental pressure which leads to obstruction of the airway by the tongue. Oral pharyngeal airways help to displace the tongue. Infants have a relatively high and anterior larynx with a U-shaped, floppy epiglottis. The use of straight laryngoscope blade facilitates exposure of the glottic opening by allowing the epiglottis to be picked up. The pediatric trachea is classically described as being conical in shape with the narrowest part being at the level of the cricoid cartilage. The pediatric airway is thus susceptible to pressure injury at this point. An inappropriately large endotracheal tube can cause barotrauma leading to postoperative stridor and rarely to necrosis and chronic subglottic stenosis. An uncuffed endotracheal tube (ETT) is classically used in pediatric patients with the presence of a small leak ensuring that the endotracheal tube is not too large. Modern cuffed ETTs are purpose-designed for pediatric patients. They have a low-pressure, high-volume cuff and can be used safely in infants and children if cuff pressure is monitored and maintained below 20 cm $H_2O$. However, the routine use of cuffed tubes cannot be justified and they are reserved for specific situations, for example, where endotracheal tube changes need to be kept to a minimum, when greater protection of the lungs from soiling is required, or when a leak around the ETT needs to be minimized.

Functional residual capacity (FRC) is the amount of air left in the lungs at the end of a normal tidal breath. The FRC acts as a reservoir for gas exchange. In infants and small children, the ratio of alveolar ventilation to FRC is twice that in an adult. The wash in and wash out of inhaled gases including oxygen is therefore rapid in infants. In practical terms, this means that changes in depth of anesthesia with inhaled agents occurs more rapidly. It also means that small children desaturate rapidly during periods of apnea. Infants and children are more reliant on diaphragmatic movement and accessory muscles rather than rib elastic recoil and rib elevation for ventilation and maintenance of FRC. The muscles of the diaphragm in infants are less resistant to fatigue (Hillier et al. 2004) and thus spontaneous ventilation under anesthesia without support is less well tolerated. Raised intra-abdominal pressure as might occur from gastric distension, laparoscopic surgery, surgical retraction, or intra-abdominal sepsis can splint the diaphragm resulting in impaired ventilation. Under general anesthesia, small airway collapse and de-recruitment of alveoli occur due to a reduction in muscle tone and activity. Infants therefore benefit from positive end-expiratory pressure (PEEP) to maintain lung volume and optimal ventilation while under anesthesia.

Neonates, and in particular premature infants, are at risk of apnea in the postoperative period due to immaturity of the respiratory control center. This risk is significantly reduced when the premature infant has reached a postmenstrual age of 54 weeks and the term infant has reached a postmenstrual age of 46 weeks. Anemia and hypothermia are additional risk factors for apnea in the newborn. If general anesthesia is necessary in infants below these ages, apnea monitoring should occur for a minimum of 12 apnea free hours. This will usually necessitate an overnight bed stay even for minor surgery.

## Cardiovascular

Neonates have what is known as a "transitional" circulation. At birth functional closure of the ductus arteriosus and the foramen ovale occurs. The pulmonary and systemic circulations are converted from two parallel systems to a circulation in series. Anatomical closure of the foramen ovale occurs between 3 months and 1 year (Hillier et al. 2004) and that of the ductus arteriosus occurs at around 2 months of age (Hillier et al. 2004). The initial functional nature of this closure means that under certain circumstances, reversal of flow can occur through the foramen ovale and the ductus arteriosus resulting in reversion to a fetal circulation with right to left shunting. This can occur if there is an increase in pulmonary vascular resistance due to hypoxemia, hypercarbia, or acidosis. As blood bypasses the lungs, hypoxemia, hypercarbia, and acidosis get worse and pulmonary vascular resistance increases. This vicious cycle with persistent pulmonary hypertension can be seen in conditions such as diaphragmatic hernia or respiratory distress syndrome (Hillier et al. 2004).

Neonates and infants have a high cardiac output to satisfy their metabolic demand for oxygen. The contractile elements of the neonatal myocardium are not fully developed. Neonates have limited ability to increase contractility and stroke volume and are therefore reliant on heart rate to maintain cardiac output. At the same time, the infant's cardiovascular system is parasympathetic dominant with an immature sympathetic nervous system. This makes them more prone to vagal responses and bradycardia can occur with hypoxemia and stimuli such as oropharyngeal suction. They have a resting heart rate that is fast, leaving little reserve. They have a poor vasoconstrictor response to hypotension and hypovolemia. Neonates and infants therefore tolerate bradycardia and even modest hypovolemia poorly. The negative inotropic and vasodilator effects of commonly used anesthetic agents are also poorly tolerated and must be anticipated. These effects can be exacerbated by positive pressure ventilation, which reduces venous return (Hillier et al. 2004).

## Fluid and Electrolytes and Blood

Neonates have a higher total body water volume, higher extracellular fluid volume, and greater water turnover when compared to adults or older children. The glomerular filtration rate is reduced in neonates and there is a reduced capacity to reabsorb sodium (Hillier et al. 2004). Hemoglobin in the neonate reaches a physiological nadir at 3 months of age. Neonates do not make antibodies to red blood cell antigens until 3 or 4 months of age. This occurs in response to bacterial colonization of the intestine. However, their plasma may contain maternal antibodies to ABO antigens. Blood transfusion in this age group uses blood that is compatible with the infant's blood type and with any maternal antibodies that may be present. ABO-compatible FFP, cryoprecipitate, and platelets should be used as incompatible units may contain sufficient antibodies to cause significant hemolysis of red blood cells. Repeated blood typing to check for newly formed antibodies is not required in the first 3–4 months of life so long as strict safety guidelines are followed. In immune compromised patients such as premature infants, blood components need to be irradiated to prevent transfusion-associated graft-versus-host disease, which occurs when transfused lymphocytes proliferate.

## Pharmacology

The principal pharmacokinetic parameters that determine the body's handling of a drug are its volume of distribution, protein binding, and elimination. These parameters all change with age and maturation. Infants and neonates have a greater proportion of extracellular fluid compared to adults. The volume of distribution for water-soluble drugs is therefore greater in infants compared to adults. As a result, bolus dosing, which is determined principally by the volume of distribution, may be greater in infants and neonates (Kemper et al. 2011; Anderson 2011). For example neonates require three times the adult dose of the commonly used muscle relaxant suxamethonium.

Some drugs have significant plasma protein binding with the pharmacodynamic effect being due to the amount of unbound drug. In neonates, alpha 1-acid glycoprotein levels are low (up to 1/3 adults) leading to a high unbound fraction of drugs such as local anesthetics and fentanyl. Alpha 1-acid glycoprotein is also an acute phase protein whose levels increase in the postoperative period due to surgical stress. Local anesthetics with a low hepatic extraction ratio may therefore exhibit a time-dependent change in clearance in the postoperative period creating a possibility of toxicity even with seemingly appropriate doses (Mazoit 2006).

Elimination occurs by metabolism in the liver and or excretion by the kidneys. Renal function is not fully developed at birth. Glomerular filtration of the kidney reaches its peak between 6 and 12 months after birth (Kemper et al. 2011). Hepatic enzyme function also continues to mature after birth. Phase I and phase II hepatic metabolism of many drugs is therefore reduced in the neonate. Infants may be more sensitive to the effects of drugs and toxic by-products. For example, the blood–brain barrier is not fully developed at birth. It is for this reasons that infants suffer kernicterus at plasma bilirubin levels that would not cause neurological effects in adults.

Pharmacodynamics, the physiological effects of drugs on the target organ, can also be age dependent. Minimum alveolar concentration (MAC) is the alveolar concentration of volatile anesthetic agent that abolishes the response to a standard skin incision in 50 % of subjects. It is used as a measure of anesthetic potency and effect. MAC for all commonly used volatile anesthetic agents is low in preterm infants. MAC is at its peak around 6 months of age when it is about 1.5–1.8 times the mean MAC of a 40-year-old adult (Mazoit 2006). There is an increased sensitivity to propofol and volatile anesthetics with age.

Pharmacokinetic and pharmacodynamic factors affect drug dosing in pediatric patients and in particular in neonates. Drug doses may need to be reduced and the dosing interval increased. Some drugs may require additional monitoring in the neonate to take into account altered distribution, metabolism, and clearance rates.

# Preoperative

## Preoperative Assessment

Surgical and anesthesia-related morbidity and mortality can be reduced by the preoperative identification of at-risk patients. Careful history and examination should allow the identification of patients at risk, and these patients should be referred for preanesthetic assessment prior to surgery. The American Society of Anesthesiologists physical status classification (ASA) was developed to describe the physical status of patients prior to surgery (Malviya et al. 2011; American Society of Anesthesiologists 1963; Saklad 1941) (see Table 2.1).

While it is not designed to predict perioperative risk, it has been found to be predictive of escalation of care, hospital admission, length of stay, and prevalence of adverse events and mortality (Malviya et al. 2011). A recent study into its use in pediatric patients has found it to be a valid and reliable tool (Malviya et al. 2011). However, it does not take into account the nature and extent of surgery and its potential effect on the patient.

**Table 2.1** American Society of Anesthesiologists Physical Status Classification (ASA). Reproduced with permission, excerpted from http://www.asahq.org/Home/For-Members/Clinical-Information/ASA-Physical-Status-Classification-System, 2013, of the American Society of Anesthesiologists. A copy of the full text can be obtained from ASA, 520 N. Northwest Highway, Park Ridge, Illinois, 60068-2573, USA

ASA 1. A normal healthy patient

ASA 2. A patient with mild systemic disease

ASA 3. A patient with severe systemic disease

ASA 4. A patient with severe systemic disease that is a constant threat to life

ASA 5. A moribund patient not expected to survive for 24 h with or without the operation

ASA 6. Declared brain-dead patient whose organs are being removed for donor purposes

A modifier "E" can be added for emergency cases

Most anesthesia-related morbidity is respiratory in nature. There is an increased incidence of respiratory adverse events in children who have a current or recent upper respiratory tract infection (URTI). Complications include bronchospasm, laryngospasm, desaturation, coughing, and stridor. It is clear that children with current severe URTI, systemic illness or signs of lower respiratory tract infection should have elective surgery postponed. A high risk of perioperative adverse events is present in the first 2 weeks after a URTI (Von Ungern-Sternberg et al. 2010). Children with URTI greater than 2 weeks prior to surgery have a low risk of perioperative respiratory events, and surgery can be undertaken. As children have six or more URTI a year, it is difficult to find a window of opportunity when they are free of URTI. For children with mild current or mild recent URTI less than 2 weeks prior to surgery, it may be appropriate to proceed for practical reasons. This approach accepts that there is an increased risk of adverse respiratory complications. Other risk factors for perioperative respiratory complications include underlying asthma, chronic lung disease of prematurity, or other chronic lung disease such as cystic fibrosis. Atopy, a strong family history of atopy, and exposure to second-hand smoking have also been found to be associated with increased risk (Von Ungern-Sternberg et al. 2010). For these children respiratory function should be optimized prior to elective surgery, and a lower threshold for postponing surgery in the presence of a URTI should be exercised. In particular, asthma should be well controlled before surgery. In children with underlying cardiac disease or chronic lung disease of prematurity, a more conservative approach is warranted as even minor respiratory complications can have potentially catastrophic consequences.

Any decision whether or not to proceed when a child has a URTI needs to involve informed consent with the parents as well as discussion with the surgeon. Other factors such as the age of the child and the nature and urgency of the surgery need to be considered. The threshold for cancellation may need to be lower in hospitals that do not look after pediatric patients on a regular basis or that do not have backup to manage complications. Anesthesia management should be tailored to minimize risk. An anesthetist with ongoing experience in pediatric anesthesia is important in minimizing risk. See Table 2.2.

**Table 2.2** Guide to preoperative decision making in the child with a URTI

| Clinical presentation | Child with no underlying cardiac or respiratory disease | Child with underlying cardiac or respiratory disease |
|---|---|---|
| Current severe URTI | Postpone for 2–3 weeks | Postpone for 4–6 weeks |
| LRTI | | |
| Fever or other signs of systemic illness | | |
| Current mild URTI | Proceed with caution[a] | Postpone for 2–4 weeks |
| URTI <2 weeks prior to surgery | | |
| URTI >2 weeks prior to surgery | Proceed | Proceed with caution or Postpone until 4 weeks after symptoms resolve |

[a]Note: Recommended for experienced anesthetist, experienced anesthetic assistant, and PACU staff. *Other factors such as the age of the child and the nature and urgency of the surgery need to be considered*

Children with congenital heart disease are another group at risk of cardiorespiratory complications in the perioperative period. This group should be referred for review. Echocardiography should be sought to assess ventricular systolic and diastolic function, intracardiac shunts, valvular dysfunction, and pulmonary hypertension. The child with a previously undiagnosed murmur presents a different challenge. Generally, children with asymptomatic murmurs who are active and keep up with their peers without shortness of breath, fatigue, cyanosis, and without difficulty feeding or failure to thrive (infants) will tolerate general anesthesia for minor surgery. Any children who are symptomatic or undergoing major surgery should be reviewed prior to surgery. All children with high-grade murmurs, diastolic murmurs, or pansystolic murmurs should also be reviewed prior to surgery. Other signs, such as reduced femoral pulses or signs of cardiac failure should be sought. Consideration should be given to indications for antibiotic prophylaxis in children with cardiac lesions.

Underlying syndromes can present multiple challenges for anesthesia. These include airway anomalies, respiratory disease, and cardiac, musculoskeletal, and renal abnormalities. A group of syndromes are associated with difficult airway and difficult intubation. These include Pierre Robin sequence, Treacher Collins syndrome, Beckwith-Wiedemann syndrome, the mucopolysaccharidoses (e.g., Hunter syndrome, Hurler syndrome, Sanfilippo syndrome), and Goldenhar syndrome, also known as Oculo-Auriculo-Vertebral (OAV) syndrome. Characteristic airway features of many of these syndromes are small mouth opening, small and recessed mandible, and a relatively large tongue. In the mucopolysaccharidoses, tissue deposits in the airway and elsewhere increase over time such that the airway becomes progressively more difficult to manage. Many syndromes have associated congenital cardiac anomalies which may or may not have required surgery. Neuromuscular and musculoskeletal abnormalities can present challenges for vascular access and positioning. Abnormalities involving the chest wall can result in restrictive lung defect and respiratory failure. Bulbar dysfunction can lead to swallowing difficulties and a tendency to recurrent aspiration further compromising respiratory function. Generalized muscle weakness or myopathy leads to sensitivity to the respiratory depressant effects of sedative, anesthetic, and analgesic agents. Some patients may require postoperative ventilation, or noninvasive respiratory support, or at the very least continuous pulse oximetry and apnea monitoring.

Malignant hyperthermia (MH) is an autosomal dominant pharmacogenetic condition. When susceptible patients are exposed to suxamethonium and volatile anesthetic agents, a hypermetabolic cascade commences in skeletal muscle. This results in rhabdomyolysis, hyperthermia, and lactic acidosis with hypercarbia. The condition is often fatal when not recognized and treated promptly. Genetic testing will provide a diagnosis in 50 % of cases (Ungern-Sternberg and Habre 2007). In vitro contracture testing of muscle biopsy is the diagnostic test. However, this can only be performed in older children because of the size of the muscle biopsy required. A trigger-free anesthetic should be used in all patients with a diagnosis of MH or with a family history of MH. Central core disease, multi-minicore disease, nemaline rod myopathy, Evan's myopathy, and King-Denborough syndrome are associated with malignant hyperthermia (MH). The muscular dystrophies (Duchenne muscular dystrophy and Becker dystrophy) can result in rhabdomyolysis with exposure to volatile anesthetic agents and suxamethonium. Hyperkalemic cardiac arrest can result. Volatile anesthetic agents should be avoided or used with extreme caution in these patients. Suxamethonium is contraindicated.

## *Fasting*

Preoperative fasting is necessary to minimize the risk of aspiration of gastric contents under anesthesia. Clear fluids will typically empty from the stomach in less than 1 h (Splinter and Schreiner 1999). Solids empty more slowly from the stomach and the rate of emptying is dependent on the volume and type of food ingested. Solids are foods that are in a solid state when in the stomach. Milk and infant formula are in a liquid form when ingested but form solid curds upon reaching the stomach (Splinter and Schreiner 1999). In general, breast milk empties faster than infant formula but nevertheless requires more than 2 h to ensure complete emptying (Splinter and Schreiner 1999). Gastric transit time is generally greater for infants than it is for adults. Factors that slow gastric emptying include trauma, pain, opiates, gastrointestinal illness, gastroesophageal reflux, and systemic illness. Studies have shown that there is unlikely to be an increase in residual gastric fluid volume in obese children after a 2-h clear fluid fast (Scott et al. 2009).

Fasting times for infants are adjusted according to their age, feeding requirements, and expected increased gastric transit time as well as according to the type of feed they ingest. There is no evidence that prolonged fasting reduces the risk of aspiration of gastric contents. Prolonged daytime fasting may increase the risk of intraoperative hypoglycemia (Leelanukrom and Cunliffe 2000). Fasting has been liberalized and clear fluids are allowed up to 2 h preoperatively in all patients

**Table 2.3** Fasting guidelines for infants and children

| |
|---|
| *Neonate and infants under 6 months* |
| Clear fluids – 2 h |
| Breast milk – 3 h |
| Formula – 4 h |
| *Infants 6 months to 12 months* |
| Clear fluids – 2 h |
| Breast milk – 4 h |
| Formula – 6 h |
| Solids – 6 h |
| *Children* |
| Clear fluids – 2 h |
| Milk – 6 h |
| Solids – 6 h |

Note: These may need modification for specific situations, patients, and procedures

without risk factors for gastric stasis. This improves patient comfort and avoids preoperative dehydration without increasing the volume or acidity of gastric contents (Splinter and Schreiner 1999; Castillo-zamora et al. 2005; Murat and Dubois 2008). While some guidelines recommend a 3-h fast after breast milk ingestion, a more conservative 4-h fast ensures low residual gastric fluid volumes in all healthy infants without causing prolonged, unnecessary distress. See Table 2.3.

## Preoperative Anxiety

It is common for children and parents to be apprehensive during the lead-up to surgery. Excessive apprehension prior to anesthesia and surgery can make the task of preparation, transfer, and anesthesia difficult and traumatic for the child and all concerned. High levels of anxiety can result in parental dissatisfaction, increased postoperative pain and analgesic requirements (Chorney and Kain 2010), and negative behavioral changes (nightmares, separation anxiety, eating problems, and increased fear of doctors) in the postoperative period. Young age is a risk factor for preoperative anxiety with preschool children between the ages of 1 and 5 being at highest risk. High baseline anxiety and previous stressful experiences with healthcare providers and high levels of parental anxiety are also predictive of preoperative anxiety. The two main methods for managing anxiety at the time of induction are sedative premedications and parental presence at induction of anesthesia. Other methods, including behavioral modification and preparation programs, may be effective but are time consuming and generally less practical.

Parental presence at induction reduces separation anxiety and is overwhelmingly preferred by parents. However, some studies have shown that while a calm parent can reduce anxiety in an anxious child, anxious parents do not benefit anxious children (Kain et al. 2006) and can lead to increased anxiety in previously calm children. The decision of whether or not to have parents present at the time of induction should be made with discussion between anesthetist and parents. The use of induction rooms allows induction of anesthesia to occur in a less threatening environment. Parents can be allowed to accompany children into the induction room or operating theater. Parental presence requires that a designated person be available to assist parents and accompany them from the operating theater or induction room once their child is anesthetized.

Sedative premedications have been found to be superior to parental presence at reducing preoperative anxiety. Midazolam and clonidine given orally are two commonly used sedative agents. Midazolam has the advantages of having a rapid onset of effect and providing sedative anxiolysis with retrograde amnesia. It has the disadvantages of being bitter to taste and a relatively short duration with peak effect after oral dosing between 20 and 30 min. Oral clonidine has no unpleasant taste. It provides sedation within 30–45 min. Clonidine is analgesic and anxiolytic but does not cause amnesia. Ketamine given orally or intramuscularly is also used as a sedative premedication. All children who have received sedative premedication should have appropriate monitoring and supervision instituted. Supplemental oxygen and continuous pulse oximetry may be required.

# Intraoperative

## *Mode of Anesthesia Induction*

Children can safely undergo inhalational or intravenous induction of anesthesia.

Inhalational induction is indicated in cases where spontaneous ventilation needs to be maintained such as difficult airway, foreign body in the airway or acute airway obstruction. Intravenous induction is indicated in the patient at risk of aspiration of gastric contents who needs a rapid sequence induction or in a child who requires resuscitation prior to induction of anesthesia. Aside from these specific indications, the choice of inhalational or intravenous induction is largely determined by the preference or experience of the anesthetist. Inhalational induction is commonly used in pediatric practice. Infants and small children may be difficult to cannulate and inhalational induction is perceived to be less threatening. It is often preferred by younger children. However, it still requires a cooperative child. It can be more distressing to achieve inhalational induction in a noncooperative child than it is to secure intravenous access. With the use of topical anesthetic preparations and skilled distraction techniques, intravenous access can be achieved in the awake child with minimal discomfort or distress. Intravenous induction is often preferred by older children. The advantages of intravenous induction include rapid onset and the inherent safety of having a cannula in place prior to loss of consciousness and loss of protective airway reflexes. Intravenous induction with propofol, the most common agent, can cause pain at the site of injection, which can be distressing and explicitly recalled.

## Patient Positioning

The size of the pediatric patient creates challenges for vascular access, placement of monitoring, patient positioning, and surgical access. Patient positioning is a team effort and should result in easy access to the airway and intravenous lines as well as allow unencumbered surgery while protecting the patient from pressure trauma and heat loss. The child is usually placed at head-end of the operating table. For small children this means that only the upper end of the table is used, so that anesthetic, surgical, and nursing staff are all clustered around one end of the table. The surgical site(s) and the airway or intravenous access sites are often very close together. This carries the risk of inadvertent dislodgment of tubes or lines, accidental de-sterilization of the operative field, and accidental injury to limbs, face, and other body parts, through pressure, retraction, or other mechanisms. Careful attention to fixing cannulae, drains, and catheters is essential. Taping of urinary catheters to the abdomen instead of the thigh reduces the risk of inadvertent (or intentional) distraction, removal, and disconnection.

## Fluid Management

Intraoperative fluid management aims to replace fasting deficit, to provide maintenance fluid to meet metabolic requirements, and to replace intraoperative losses. Fasting deficit can easily be calculated by multiplying the hourly maintenance fluid requirements by the number of hours fasted. This fluid can be replaced over the duration of the procedure for long cases (Leelanukrom and Cunliffe 2000). An alternative approach is to administer 25 ml/kg to replace routine fasting deficit in children up to 3 years of age and 15 ml/kg in children 4 years and over (Leelanukrom and Cunliffe 2000). If intravenous fluids have been commenced preoperatively, this may not be necessary. Modifications may need to be made in situations where there is increased loss or deficit such as febrile illness or sepsis. The acutely hypovolemic child should be resuscitated prior to induction of anesthesia. Induction of anesthesia in a hypovolemic patient can lead to catastrophic hypotension and even cardiac arrest. Maintenance requirements in the anesthetized child are minimal and 4 ml/kg/h provides a reasonable guide. Insensible loss can be as high as 20 ml/kg/h for major abdominal surgery or up to 50 ml/kg/h during procedures with high exposure and high third space losses such as necrotizing enterocolitis or repair of gastroschisis in premature infants (Leelanukrom and Cunliffe 2000; Murat and Dubois 2008). See Table 2.4.

Estimating fluid loss and volume state can be difficult and may necessitate invasive monitoring and serial arterial blood gas analysis to measure lactate, electrolytes, and hemoglobin. A precordial stethoscope is a useful noninvasive adjunct and relies on changes in heart sounds with rapid changes in volume state. Communication between the surgeon and anesthetist is important in anticipating and managing loss. Insensible losses, including third space losses, should be replaced intraoperatively

**Table 2.4** Guide schedule for fluid replacement in children

|  | Rate | Reference(s) |
|---|---|---|
| *Fasting deficit replacement fluids* | | |
| Children up to 3 years of age | 25 ml/kg | Murat and Dubois (2008) |
| Children 4 years and over | 15 ml/kg | Murat and Dubois (2008) |
| *Maintenance fluids* | | |
| Intraoperative | 4 ml/kg/h | Murat and Dubois (2008) |
| *Insensible intraoperative losses* | | |
| Minor surgery | 2–10 ml/kg/h | Murat and Dubois (2008) |
| Major surgery (abdominal, thoracic) | 15–20 ml/kg/h | Leelanukrom and Cunliffe (2000) |
| *Blood* | | |
| Replace estimated losses | 1:1 with blood or colloid | Leelanukrom and Cunliffe (2000), Murat and Dubois (2008) |
|  | 3:1 with crystalloid | |

with crystalloid up to 30–50 ml/kg (Murat and Dubois 2008). Beyond this it is appropriate to change to a colloid to maintain oncotic pressure particularly in those who are susceptible to pulmonary and peripheral edema. Albumin is the main colloid used for volume expansion in neonates and infants (Murat and Dubois 2008). Blood loss should be replaced on a 1:1 basis with colloid and 3:1 basis with crystalloid.

Hypoglycemia in otherwise healthy children who have not been subject to a prolonged fast is rare (Leelanukrom and Cunliffe 2000). Neonates have decreased glycogen stores and a reduced capacity for gluconeogenesis (Leelanukrom and Cunliffe 2000). They are therefore susceptible to hypoglycemia, with neonates less than 48 h and preterm infants being more susceptible. Regional anesthesia reduces the stress response to surgery and may result in lower blood sugar levels (Leelanukrom and Cunliffe 2000). Other risk factors include poor nutritional status and maternal diabetes. A practical method would be to run a maintenance glucose-containing solution for susceptible patients at a rate sufficient to prevent hypoglycemia (Leelanukrom and Cunliffe 2000). The use of glucose-containing solutions can result in hyperglycemia, diuresis, dehydration, and electrolyte imbalance. Hyperglycemia can also increase the risk of hypoxic, ischemic brain and spinal cord injury in susceptible patients (Leelanukrom and Cunliffe 2000; Murat and Dubois 2008). Monitoring of blood glucose levels may be necessary in infants susceptible to hypoglycemia or hyperglycemia.

## Blood Transfusion

Children have a higher incidence of adverse events related to blood transfusion when compared to adults. A recent UK audit of transfusion practice in pediatrics found that children had an adverse event rate of 18 per 100,000 transfusions compared to the adult rate of 13:100,000 (Harrison and Bolton 2011). The adverse event rate for children under 1 year was 37 per 100,000 transfusions (Harrison and Bolton 2011). A common cause of incompatible transfusion is laboratory error. This may reflect the complexity of transfusion in this age group (Harrison and Bolton 2011). Inappropriate transfusion, usually over transfusion, also occurs commonly. Administrative errors may occur more frequently in neonates who may not have been named or have a name change and in any children who cannot confirm their identity. Other common errors include failure to use leukocyte-depleted blood or CMV-negative blood in children under 1 (Harrison and Bolton 2011). Acute transfusion reactions are the most common non-error-related complications in the overall pediatric population (Harrison and Bolton 2011). Electrolyte disturbance leading to arrhythmia is a real risk for neonates and infants receiving blood transfusions. Irradiation increases potassium leak out of stored red cells. Hypocalcemia occurs in response to citrated plasma. Neonates have a reduced ability to metabolize citrate. They have lower ionized calcium stores and have a myocardium that is more dependent on ionized calcium for its function. Hypothermia from rapid transfusion of cold blood also increases the risk of arrhythmia. Dilutional coagulopathy and toxicity from additives can occur with massive transfusion. Transfusion transmitted infections are rare with bacterial contamination accounting for more than 2/3 of cases (Lavoie 2011). Transfusion-related acute lung injury (TRALI) is rare in children (Lavoie 2011).

Safe transfusion in this population requires an understanding of the specific requirements of neonates and infants, standardized prescription methods to avoid over transfusion, and strict methods of checking and crosschecking to avoid administrative errors. Blood transfusion should be guided by the measured hemoglobin and by the degree of ongoing bleeding.

# Postoperative

## Intravenous Fluid Management

Historically, hypotonic fluids have been prescribed to children as maintenance following the "4, 2, 1" rule described by Holliday and Segar in 1957 (Holliday and Segar 1957). However, there is now overwhelming evidence that hypotonic solutions should not be administered routinely to children as there is a risk of hyponatremic encephalopathy, permanent brain damage, and death (Murat and Dubois 2008; Moritz and Ayus 2011). Most deaths and neurological injury due to hyponatremia occur in the postsurgical setting (Moritz and Ayus 2007). In the postoperative period, multiple non-osmotic factors lead to an increase in the release of antidiuretic hormone (ADH) resulting in free water retention. These include volume depletion, the stress response to surgery, pain, nausea, and vomiting. Pulmonary pathology and intracranial pathology or surgery can also lead to increased release of ADH (Moritz and Ayus 2011; Moritz and Ayus 2007). When hypotonic solutions are administered in the postoperative setting, hyponatremia can occur rapidly.

Where possible, children should be allowed oral fluid intake within the first 3 h postoperatively (Murat and Dubois 2008). After major surgery, where there is a risk of elevated ADH, maintenance fluids should be decreased by 1/3 for the first day postoperatively so long as the patient is normovolemic. The ideal postoperative maintenance solution in terms of maintaining fluid and electrolyte balance as well as providing sufficient dextrose to meet energy demands is the subject of current research. What is clear is that hypotonic solutions should be avoided as maintenance. Ongoing losses should be replaced by either lactated ringers solution or normal saline. While hypoglycemia is clearly harmful, hyperglycemia is also associated with complications including exacerbation of hypoxic ischemic insult in at-risk children (Murat and Dubois 2008). Solutions containing less than 5 % dextrose are now under investigation (Moritz and Ayus 2007). Electrolyte and glucose concentrations should be monitored daily in all patients receiving intravenous fluid replacement.

## Pain Management

Until relatively recently, it was believed that neonates did not have the necessary development to perceive pain. It is now recognized that neurological and endocrine development is mature enough for pain perception prior to birth. Term and preterm infants perceive pain and display a stress response that can be measured by increases in stress hormone levels (Hillier et al. 2004). In fact neonates may have increased sensitivity to painful stimuli because of relative immaturity of descending inhibitory pathways (Ghai et al. 2008). Moreover, pain has been shown to have deleterious effects on neonates increasing morbidity and mortality (Mancuso and Burns 2009). The goal of postoperative analgesia in pediatric patients is to provide safe, effective pain relief with as few side effects as possible (Howard et al. 2008). An analgesic plan should be arranged prior to surgery and wherever possible should involve discussion between the patient, parents or caregivers, surgeon, and anesthetist. Assessment of pain is critical in effective pain management. Assessment of pain in infants and small children is reliant on monitoring physiological parameters and age-appropriate behavioral indicators. These can be standardized into objective scales such as the Children's Hospital of Eastern Ontario Pain Scale (CHEOPS) suitable for ages 1–18 and the Premature Infant Pain Profile (PIPP) (Howard et al. 2008). Older children are able to report pain and pain scores using modified visual analogue and numerical rating scores. An acute pain management service experienced in assessing and managing pediatric pain allows regular, standardized assessment and documentation of pain and analgesic modalities. This has been shown to contribute to the prevention and relief of pain improving efficacy and safety (Howard et al. 2008).

The full range of analgesic modalities used in adults can be used in pediatric patients. Regional anesthesia and analgesia techniques are generally done in anesthetized or heavily sedated pediatric patients. Regional analgesic techniques include peripheral nerve blocks with or without a continuous infusion catheter. Caudal, lumbar, and thoracic epidural blocks with or without catheter placement are also used. Neuraxial local anesthetic blocks can be prolonged or augmented by the use of adjuvants such as opioids, clonidine (alpha agonist), and preservative-free ketamine. Single shot caudal epidural blocks are extremely effective for many procedures below the level of the umbilicus. This simple block has an excellent safety profile and a low failure rate (Howard et al. 2008). The use of ultrasound has improved the safety and efficacy of many regional techniques.

Parenteral analgesics such as opioids and ketamine can be administered by continuous infusion, patient-controlled analgesia (PCA), or by nurse-controlled analgesia. Pediatric oral opioid preparations are available allowing for flexible oral analgesic regimes to be implemented either as sole strategy or as a step-down from parenteral analgesia. Adjuvant analgesics include paracetamol, tramadol, NSAIDs, and clonidine. Antispasmodics such as baclofen and diazepam are useful in some settings.

## Postoperative Nausea and Vomiting

Postoperative nausea and vomiting (PONV) is estimated to occur in 20–30 % of the general surgical population and in up to 70–80 % of high-risk patients (Gan et al. 2007). Rates of PONV may be higher in pediatric patients. PONV is distressing. Studies have indicated that adults ranked emesis as the most undesirable postoperative complication above pain which was ranked third (Gan 2006). In addition, PONV can increase length of stay in the postanesthesia care unit and can lead to overnight admission in patients who would otherwise been appropriate for day of surgery discharge. Anesthesia-related independent risk factors for PONV are general anesthesia with volatile anesthetics, nitrous oxide, and the use of intraoperative and postoperative opioids (Gan et al. 2007). Avoiding or minimizing the use of these agents will reduce the baseline risk for PONV. In addition, there is good evidence to show that adequate hydration also reduces the risk of PONV (Gan et al. 2007). Independent risk factors for postoperative vomiting in children include duration of surgery (greater than 30 min), age greater than 3 years, strabismus surgery, and a positive history of postoperative vomiting in the patient, a sibling, or a parent (Gan et al. 2007). The risk of postoperative vomiting is increased when more of these independent risk factors were present (Gan et al. 2007). Prophylactic antiemetic therapy has been shown to reduce the incidence of PONV in children and should be administered to all children with an increased risk of PONV (Gan et al. 2007). Combination therapy is more effective than mono therapy. Drugs that can be used for anti emetic prophylaxis in children include 5-HT3 receptor antagonists, dexamethasone, droperidol, promethazine, and metoclopramide. In patients with established postoperative vomiting who have received prophylaxis, an antiemetic from a different class should be used. If no prophylaxis has been given, then a 5-HT3 receptor antagonist should be given.

## Emergence Delirium

Emergence delirium (ED), also known as emergence agitation, refers to behavioral disturbance that occurs following general anesthesia. ED has an incidence of 20–30 % and is most common among preschool-aged children (Vlajkovic and Sindjelic 2007). It is characterized by agitation, confusion, hallucinations, and restlessness or thrashing (Bajwa et al. 2010). Children do not recognize family members and do not make eye contact with caregivers. The cause of ED is unclear. It occurs in the immediate postoperative period usually in the postanesthesia care unit. ED was thought to be secondary to rapid awakening after anesthesia with newer shorter acting inhaled anesthetic agents such as sevoflurane. ED occurs more commonly with certain types of surgery including squint surgery and ear nose and throat surgery (Vlajkovic and Sindjelic 2007). However, it does occur in children who have had a general anesthetic for a nonsurgical procedure such as an MRI scan. Emergence delirium is usually self-limiting and in most cases will resolve within the first 30 min. Children generally have no recollection of the episode. However, it is distressing to parents and can place patients at risk of injury including damage to surgical sights, drains, and cannulae. Emergence delirium can prolong stay in the postanesthesia care unit and requires increased recovery room resources to manage. The management of emergence delirium includes, protecting patients from harm, providing a quiet environment for recovery, excluding pain as a cause and reassuring family members. Agents that have been shown to reduce the duration and severity of emergence delirium include clonidine, fentanyl, propofol, and midazolam. These can be used in severe or prolonged cases. Strategies that have been used to reduce the incidence of emergence delirium in high-risk patients include premedication with oral midazolam, intravenous clonidine, dexmedetomidine, and fentanyl and the use of propofol anesthesia.

## Risks and Complications

### Morbidity

The risk of serious morbidity or death from anesthesia is extremely low in healthy children (Van der Griend et al. 2011) when they are cared for by staff experienced in pediatric anesthesia in a health-care facility experienced with looking after children. The risk of death and cardiac arrest during anesthesia is very low. The groups at greatest risk are neonates and children with cardiac disease. Children with pulmonary hypertension are at particular risk (Van der Griend et al. 2011). These children should only undergo anesthesia if surgery is absolutely unavoidable and then only in a tertiary pediatric center with experienced staff. It is important to note that nearly half the complications of anesthesia in children occur in the postanesthesia care unit (PACU) and most are respiratory or airway complications. The most common serious complication is laryngospasm where laryngeal spasm results in acute and complete airway obstruction and potentially life-threatening hypoxemia and cardiac arrest. Post-extubation stridor occurs when edema and swelling of the narrow pediatric airway lead to partial obstruction. Good outcomes require anesthetists and nursing staff both in the PACU and the ward to be thoroughly familiar with looking after children. PACU and ward staff must be able to rapidly identify a sick child and be able to manage their airway in the event of obstruction or apnea. Other complications such as emergence delirium, behavioral change, and postoperative nausea and vomiting have been described above.

## Awareness

Awareness is the explicit recall of events that occurred during anesthesia. In adults this occurs in about 0.1 % of anesthetics and is associated with significant psychological consequences in about 25 % of cases. In children awareness is more common, occurring in about 0.7 % of anesthetics. It is unknown why awareness is more common in children, but interestingly there is some evidence to suggest that the incidence of serious psychological consequences may not be as high as in adults. Nevertheless, some children do develop serious consequences so any child reporting awareness should be taken seriously and referral made for psychological follow-up and support. Psychological problems may present late so the follow-up should be ongoing.

## Effect of General Anesthesia on the Developing Brain

Children are different to adults in that many organs are still developing and hence are vulnerable to toxic insults. In particular the brain undergoes significant development after birth and throughout early childhood. There is now good evidence in animal models that general anesthetic agent causes neuronal death (apoptosis). There is also evidence in the animal model that newborn monkeys and rodents exposed to general anesthesia have later neurobehavioral problems. It is difficult to know how to translate this to the human as doses and periods of development vary from animal to human. Numerous human cohort studies do show an association between surgery in early childhood and poor neurobehavioral outcome. The association is strongest for children having major surgery in the neonatal period, though one study does show an association between multiple anesthetics in young children beyond infancy and poor outcome (Wilder et al. 2009). In all these studies, it is unclear if this association is due to the anesthesia, the surgery, or the condition which underlies the need for surgery or anesthesia. It must be noted that there is strong evidence that surgery in the neonate without adequate anesthesia and analgesia results in poor outcome. Withholding surgery or anesthesia is not an option in children that require surgery clinically. Further research is under way to try and determine the exact risk of neurotoxicity of anesthesia and to determine the optimal anesthetic to give these children. In the meantime the FDA and many other bodies recommend that purely elective surgery is avoided in infancy, because of the potential risks that anesthesia may be neurotoxic to the developing brain.

# Summary

Pediatric anesthesia presents a variety of differences when compared to adult anesthesia for surgery. Pediatric surgery is performed in preterm infants through to adult-size teenagers. Psychological development affects conduct of anesthesia and postoperative management including analgesic plans. The coexistence of other anomalies, some of which may be life threatening, often adds another layer of complexity to pediatric anesthesia and surgery. The type of anesthesia and approaches used will vary with the type of surgery and the age, "size," and "mental maturity" of the patient. This chapter describes the *anatomical, physiological, and psychological* challenges that are unique to pediatric surgery and anesthesia. Consent issues are highlighted as being vitally important. Careful preoperative assessment and good communication between anesthetist and surgeon are essential for good clinical outcomes.

**Acknowledgments** Mr. M Gorton is acknowledged with reference to the consent discussion (see Volume 1).

# Further Reading, References, and Resources

American Society of Anesthesiologists. New classification of physical status. Anesthesiology. 1963;24:111.

Anderson BJ. Developmental pharmacology; filling one knowledge gap in pediatric anesthesiology. Paediatr Anaesth. 2011;21(3):179–82.

Bajwa SA, Costi D, Cyna AM. A comparison of emergence delirium scales following general anesthesia in children. Pediatr Anesth. 2010;20:704–11.

Castillo-zamora C, et al. Randomized trial comparing overnight preoperative fasting period vs oral administration of apple juice at 06:00–06:30 AM in pediatric orthopedic surgical patients. Paediatr Anesth. 2005;15:638–42.

Chorney JM, Kain ZN. Family-centred pediatric perioperative care. Anesthesiology. 2010;112: 751–5.

Gan TJ. Risk factors for postoperative nausea and vomiting. Anesth Analg. 2006;102:1884–98.

Gan TJ, et al. Society for ambulatory anesthesia guidelines for the management of postoperative nausea and vomiting. Anesth Analg. 2007;105:1615–28.

Ghai B, Makkar JK, Wig J. Postoperative pain assessment in preverbal children and children with cognitive impairment pediatric anesthesia (Review article). Pediatr Anesth. 2008;18:462–77.

Harrison E, Bolton P. Serious hazards of transfusion in children (SHOT). Review article. Pediatr Anesth. 2011;21:10–3.

Hillier SC, Krishna G, Brasoveanu E. Neonatal anesthesia. Semin Pediatr Surg. 2004;13(3): 142–51.

Holliday MA, Segar WE. The maintenance need for water in parenteral fluid therapy. Pediatrics. 1957;19:823–32.

Howard R, Carter B, Curry J, Morton N, Rivett K, Rose M, Tyrrell J, Walker S, Williams G; Association of Paediatric Anaesthetists of Great Britain and Ireland. Good practice in postoperative and procedural pain management. Background. Paediatr Anaesth. 2008;18 Suppl 1:1–3.

Kain ZN, et al. Predicting which child–parent pair will benefit from parental presence during induction of anesthesia: a decision-making approach. Anesth Analg. 2006;102:81–4.

Kemper EM, et al. Towards evidence-based pharmacotherapy in children. Pediatr Anesth. 2011; 21:183–9.

Lavoie J. Blood transfusion risks and alternative strategies in pediatric patients. Review article. Pediatr Anesth. 2011;21:14–24.

Leelanukrom R, Cunliffe M. Intraoperative fluid and glucose management in children. Paediatr Anaesth. 2000;10:353–9.

Malviya S, et al. Does an objective system-based approach improve assessment of perioperative risk in children? A preliminary evaluation of the 'NARCO'. Br J Anaesth. 2011;106(3): 352–8.

Mancuso T, Burns J. Ethical concerns in the management of pain in the neonate. Pediatr Anesth. 2009;19:953–7.

Mazoit JX. Pharmacokinetic/pharmacodynamic modeling of anesthetics in children. Therapeutic implications. Pediatr Drugs. 2006;8(3):140–50.

Moritz ML, Ayus JC. Hospital-acquired hyponatremia – why are hypotonic parenteral fluids still being used? Nat Clin Pract Nephrol. 2007;3(7):374–82.

Moritz ML, Ayus JC. Intravenous fluid management for the acutely ill child. Curr Opin Pediatr. 2011;23:186–93.

Murat I, Dubois M-C. Perioperative fluid therapy in pediatrics (Review article). Paediatr Anesth. 2008;18:363–70.

Saklad M. Grading of patients for surgical procedures. Anesthesiology. 1941;2:281–4.

Scott D, et al. Overweight/obesity and gastric fluid characteristics in pediatric day surgery: implications for fasting guidelines and pulmonary aspiration risk. Anesth Analg. 2009;109: 727–36.

Splinter WM, Schreiner MS. Preoperative fasting in children. Anesth Analg. 1999;89:80–9.

Van der Griend BF, et al. Postoperative mortality in children after 101,885 anesthetics at a tertiary pediatric hospital. Anesth Analg. 2011;112:1440–7.

Vlajkovic GP, Sindjelic RP. Emergence delirium in children: many questions, few answers. Anesth Analg. 2007;104:84–91.

Von Ungern-Sternberg BS, Habre W. Review article pediatric anesthesia – potential risks and their assessment: part I. Pediatr Anesth. 2007;17:206–15.

Von Ungern-Sternberg BS, Habre W. Review article pediatric anesthesia – potential risks and their assessment: part I. Pediatr Anesth. 2007;17:206–15.

Wilder RT, et al. Early exposure to anesthesia and learning disabilities in a population-based birth cohort. Anesthesiology. 2009;110(4):796–804.

# Additional Reading

Kain ZN, Caldwell-Andrews AA. Preoperative psychological preparation of the child for surgery: an update. Anesthesiol Clin North Am. 2005;23:597–614.

Sumpelmann R, et al. A novel isotonic-balanced electrolyte solution with 1 % glucose for intraoperative fluid therapy in children: results of a prospective multicentre observational postauthorization safety study (PASS). Pediatr Anesth. 2010;20:977–81.

Von Ungern-Sternberg BS, Habre W. Review article pediatric anesthesia – potential risks and their assessment: part II. Paediatr Anesth. 2007;17:311–20.

# Chapter 3
# Pediatric Abdominal Surgery

Andrew Ford, John Hutson, and Brendon J. Coventry

## General Perspective and Overview

The major difference between counseling in pediatric surgery and any other surgical specialty is that counseling is done through a third party, the parents or other significant carers/guardians. As a result, no matter what decision is made, neonates and children will be excluded from a decision that may well affect them for the rest of their lives. This is especially true when correcting major congenital anomalies in the newborn. In diaphragmatic hernia, for example, we are able to determine which fetuses may well survive, and those that are likely to die at birth, giving the parents the option of perhaps terminating the pregnancy if the lesion is discovered early enough, or even embarking on prenatal therapy. Any such counseling has to be done with caution and with many caveats, as ultrasound is not totally accurate for subtle differences from the norm. Furthermore, there may well be implications for intellectual delay in many of the fetuses with an anatomical abnormality.

The section is divided for practical purposes into (i) newborn/infant and (ii) older child. Neonates and older children often have different patterns of surgical complications. *In the newborn*, the complications of surgery are often directly related to the anatomical abnormality that has to be corrected and any associated anomalies that impact on recovery. *In the older child*, the patterns of complications are more likely to follow those seen after surgery in the younger adult, but the child is far more able

A. Ford, MB, ChB, ChM, FRCSEd, FRCS, FRACS (✉)
Division of Paediatric Surgery (Chief of Surgery), Women's and Children's Hospital,
Adelaide, Australia
e-mail: andrew.ford@me.com

J. Hutson, BS, MD, FRACS, DSc, FRAP (hon)
Department of Paediatrics, Royal Children's Hospital, Melbourne, Australia

B.J. Coventry, BMBS, PhD, FRACS, FACS, FRSM
Discipline of Surgery, Royal Adelaide Hospital, University of Adelaide,
L5 Eleanor Harrald Building, North Terrace, 5000 Adelaide, SA, Australia
e-mail: brendon.coventry@adelaide.edu.au

B.J. Coventry (ed.), *Pediatric Surgery*, Surgery: Complications, Risks and Consequences,     25
DOI 10.1007/978-1-4471-5439-6_3, © Springer-Verlag London 2014

to tolerate and recover from surgery than an adult – both physically and psychologically. This division is, of course, not absolute, and surgery usually performed in the older child may need to be performed in the newborn or infant on occasions. Likewise, surgery performed in the newborn or infant may need to be performed, or perhaps even repeated later, in the older child in special circumstances.

The *neonate* is physically primed to tolerate the massive physiological changes that occur at birth, and as a result, neonates appear to tolerate the physiological changes associated with surgery that may prove lethal to most adults (Rowe 1998). Nevertheless, their immune system is immature (Grant et al. 1997), they may have hereditary congenital diseases, and they may have anatomical anomalies that impact dramatically on the success or failure of any surgery.

Neonates with congenital anatomical anomalies often have more than one. Take, for example, esophageal atresia (an incomplete esophagus). This anatomical anomaly can be associated with anorectal abnormalities, vertebral anomalies, urinary tract anomalies, upper limb deformities, and most importantly major cardiac defects that may prove lethal (Harmon et al. 1998).

Neonates may also have underlying hereditary problems that not only predispose them to surgical problems but may also predispose them to a prolonged and complicated recovery. For example, babies with cystic fibrosis have a 14 % chance of having a small bowel obstruction at birth (meconium ileus), which will often require a laparotomy (Efrati et al. 2010). These babies may also have perforated their intestine before birth causing meconium peritonitis and massive dense adhesions (Rescorla et al. 1998) or may also have undergone an antenatal segmental volvulus. After any surgery, all babies with cystic fibrosis are at risk of progressive lung damage, which is accelerated by their requirement for a longer postoperative ventilation period than other babies.

Preterm delivery adds to the problems of any surgery and induces surgical problems of its own (Rowe 1998). Anatomical anomalies can also induce preterm labor and delivery. For example, esophageal atresia blocks swallowing and induces polyhydramnios, which in turn can trigger preterm labor. Thus, the birth weight of babies with esophageal atresia is frequently below 2.0 Kg and is often close to 1.0 Kg. Therefore, after surgery, ventilation is required which adds to the preoperative problems of gastric contents soiling the lungs from below (coming up the commonly present fistula from the stomach to the trachea) and saliva entering the lungs from above, as it cannot go down the blocked esophagus (Also see section on "Esophageal Atresia" later in this Volume).

Premature babies have diminished immune function and a very labile vascular system. When stressed a premature baby may well shut down the blood supply to the intestine and produce malfunction of the mucosal barrier in the small bowel. As a result, bacteria within the gut lumen can get into the intestinal wall and set up an active and proliferating infection. This infection is frequently with gas-producing organisms, so "gas gangrene" of the intestinal wall is the result – "necrotizing enterocolitis" (NEC) (Albanese et al. 1998). While this would appear to be a terrible situation where a tiny premature baby (some as small as 500 g) has gas gangrene of the intestinal wall, these babies respond well to antibiotics, IV feeding, and gut rest and may even survive a laparotomy with massive gut resection. This physiological insult does, however, enhance the likelihood of the extremely small premature baby having "intellectual delay" (Chacko et al. 1999) (see section on "NEC").

So, there are distinct advantages and disadvantages to carrying out surgery in the newborn period. On the whole, however, the full-term neonate responds well to surgery and survives that surgery surprisingly well; the premature may survive, but may be compromised. This improved tolerance to surgery extends to some extent into older children, so that the otherwise well child is a far better candidate for routine surgery than an adult, in general terms. The healing process is rapid, and there are rarely the psychological issues that appear to slow recovery in some adults.

But again, there are chronic diseases in the child that predispose to a poor outcome and predispose to the requirement for surgery in the first place. One common example would be cerebral palsy. These children often suffer severe intellectual delay and lie all day in contorted positions because of spasticity. They are prone to severe gastroesophageal reflux and feeding difficulties. As a result they often come to fundoplication with a gastrostomy or either one alone. But, cerebral palsy is associated with a poor outcome from that form of surgery, and there is a 30–50 % failure rate for fundoplication in this group (Boix-Ochoa et al. 1998).

Pediatric patients and surgical operations are often different from many procedures that are performed in adults, although many similarities, of course, exist. Diagnosis is frequently and increasingly within the antenatal period for a range of congenital conditions and anomalies. Even surgery is able to be performed in utero for some conditions, but many are corrected after birth. Disorders that require immediate surgery may be true emergencies or are virtually semi-elective in nature, where rapid patient optimization, or even a period of stabilization or growth, is preferable before surgery. As mentioned before, the relative *lack of ability to communicate* directly with the patient is another fundamental difference, necessitating the absolute reliance on the parent, guardian or State to make decisions on the child's part, with the advice of the surgeon, medical practitioners and other advisors.

Especially with many types of neonatal surgery, the options are extremely limited should surgery not be possible or performed, and often the natural consequence of not performing surgery is *death*. Examples of these situations are severe forms of esophageal atresia, biliary atresia, liver tumors, neuroblastoma, large congenital diaphragmatic hernia, exomphalos (also termed omphalocele), and pyloric stenosis. Despite surgery, death may still ensue.

*Parent's expectations* may not be realistic, and their individual understanding of the situation that their child is in may not be complete or even adequate to make rational and informed decisions. The situations are often emotionally charged, and the clinician(s) is always dependent on the capacity and willingness for understanding, especially in situations where the options with and without surgery are dire and carry high risks of morbidity and mortality. Realization of this must be kept in mind when medicolegal considerations are made.

The situation and available facilities are important too, as these are not equivalent for all patients in all countries throughout the world.

With these factors and facts in mind, the information given in these chapters must be appropriately and discernibly interpreted and used.

The **use of specialized units with standardized preoperative assessment, multidisciplinary input, and high-quality postoperative care** is essential to the success of complex pediatric surgery overall and can significantly reduce risk of complications or aid early detection, prompt intervention, and cost.

Many of the procedures explained here are of a more "straightforward" nature and are elective, so that the time and ability to explain to the parents and even the patient (for older children) is often more realistic and practical. In emergency settings, the ability to do this and assimilate information may be different.

**Important Note**

It should be emphasized that the risks and frequencies that are given here *represent derived figures*. These *figures are best estimates of relative frequencies across most institutions*, not merely the highest-performing ones, and as such are often representative of a number of studies, which include different patients with differing comorbidities and different surgeons. In addition, the risks of complications in lower- or higher-risk patients may lie outside these estimated ranges, and individual clinical judgment is required as to the expected risks communicated to the patient and staff or for other purposes. The range of risks is also derived from experience and the literature; while risks outside this range may exist, certain risks may be reduced or absent due to variations of procedures or surgical approaches. It is recognized that different patients, practitioners, institutions, regions, and countries may vary in their requirements and recommendations.

**Important Caveat**

The section contains a description of the more common diseases and procedures carried out in the pediatric age group, but cannot be exhaustive. There are diseases and procedures that are carried out in both children and adults, but for those that are more common in young adults, readers are referred to that section.

# Pediatric Surgery in the Newborn and Infant

## Introduction

*Abdominal wall defects in the newborn and infant* can vary from a small congenital umbilical hernia due to failure of the umbilical cicatrix to close completely by birth to major failure of the abdominal wall to develop with complete herniation of the exposed abdominal contents. The former usually closes by 2 years of age, while the larger defects may not be compatible with life, with or without surgery, especially with coexistence of other congenital anomalies. Small abdominal wall herniae are covered under the section "Pediatric Surgery in the Older Child," but may apply to surgery in the newborn and infant in certain situations where early repair is advisable. The major defects of the abdominal wall are essentially all surgically repaired early in life and are included here in this section of the chapter, although further surgical procedures may be required into childhood and adulthood. Inguinal herniae can occur at any age in the child or adult, but are especially liable to strangulate in children under 1 year of age, so are typically repaired promptly after diagnosis, so are described under this section, but may apply for the older child too.

*General abdominal surgical procedures in the newborn and infant* include a variety of procedures principally related to obstruction of the tracts of the gut or biliary systems arising from, for example, atresia, intussusception, hypertrophy, or malrotation; infections; or internal herniation. Although these are principally surgical procedures performed in the newborn and infant, they may be performed or revised in the older child also. Some of the surgical procedures described in section "Pediatric Surgery in the Older Child" may apply also to surgery in the newborn and infant in certain situations, such as gastrostomy or appendectomy.

# Pediatric Surgery in the Newborn and Infant

## *Abdominal Wall Defect Surgery*

### Open Herniotomy (Inguinal Hernia "Repair")

#### Description

Open inguinal hernia correction in children is performed under general anesthesia. Inguinal herniae occur through the anterior abdominal wall, via the deep inguinal ring, when a patent processus vaginalis persists as it follows the testicle down to the scrotum. Herniotomy is a relatively simple procedure that ligates the peritoneal sac at its origin at the deep inguinal ring and does not aim to repair the defect itself, as opposed to the aim in adult inguinal hernia repair which repairs the defective muscle wall. Because inguinal herniae in the first year of life are especially at risk of strangulation, prompt repair is advisable. In older children, unless symptomatic, elective repair within a month or two is advisable.

#### Anatomical Points

In children under one year of age, the deep and superficial inguinal rings overlie each other, and the peritoneal sac protrudes almost directly outward beneath the skin. In older children, the deep inguinal ring moves further and further laterally so that it is approximately deep to the midpoint of the inguinal ligament, so the inguinal canal is formed. This contains the spermatic cord in the male or the vestigial processus vaginalis in the female (some refer to this as the gubernaculum), and herniae arising at the deep ring transit indirectly from the deep toward the superficial opening.

It is rare for the defect to be big in the child, so that a simple herniotomy is effective. No strengthening procedure such as mesh is required. The size of the defect may be bigger in the ventilated premature; otherwise, the defect is usually small. In the male, the hernia contains bowel or omentum. In males, inguinal herniae are the most common surgical condition, usually within the first year (particularly the first 3 months) of life, with about 60 % right sided, 25 % left, and 15 % bilateral. About 12 % of all indirect inguinal herniae occur in females, where the hernia usually contains the ipsilateral ovary and the fallopian tube. Rarely the appendix (nearly always the ovary in the female) may insinuate into the sac. The testis in the neonatal male may not have descended properly, making it necessary to do an orchidopexy at the same time, so as to avoid scar tissue holding the testicle up and making subsequent orchidopexy very difficult.

It is important to realize that in the child, the gonad is at risk of infarction. The testis in the male due to incarcerated bowel presses on the testicular veins, and in the female, the ovary and tube can tort on their long axis. It is also important to realize that the younger the child, the smaller the ring(s), the more likely it is that the bowel will incarcerate and therefore put the gonad at risk. Therefore, the younger the child presents with a hernia, the sooner the surgery should be done. In the newborn, this should be within days. There is no place for the "wait until the child is older and bigger for the surgery" approach.

**Perspective**

See Table 3.1. Herniotomy is a much simpler procedure than open inguinal hernia repair in adults. Complications from herniotomy are infrequent and usually minor in nature. However, precise recording of these is limited by under-reporting. Spermatic cord injury occurs in at least 1 in 200 children (as the histopathology of the resected sac does not take into account internal blockage of the vas from handling). Therefore, the practice of exploring both sides in males under 2–4 years of age is disappearing. Bowel injury is rare, but when it does occur in the compromised ventilated neonate, it can trigger necrotizing enterocolitis and major ongoing problems. Infection and bleeding are other complications, but are usually minor. True recurrence rates are not known, as the follow-up must extend into later adult life to accurately analyze these, and most patients are lost to late follow-up. But, within childhood, the recurrence rate for healthy children could be as low as 0.1 % for open surgery and 3–5 % for laparoscopic closure of the deep ring, thereby implying that laparoscopic closure has a greatly increased recurrence rate in children. In the male, an asynchronous hernia occurs in approximately 8 % on the right if the index (initial) hernia repair was on the left and 4 % on the left if the previous

**Table 3.1** Open herniotomy (inguinal hernia "repair") estimated frequency of complications, risks, and consequences

| Complications, risks, and consequences | Estimated frequency |
|---|---|
| *Most significant/serious complications* | |
| Bleeding or hematoma formation[a] | 1–5 % |
| Hernia recurrence[a] (10 year) | |
|   For open surgery | 0.1–1 % |
|   For laparoscopic surgery | 1–5 % |
| Testicular ischemia, testicular atrophy | |
|   Incarcerated, but forcibly reducible | 1–5 % |
|   Incarcerated, but forcibly not reducible | 5–20 % |
| Ovarian torsion/loss (ovarian loss in the newborn has been reported to be up to 14 %) | 5–20 % |
| Small bowel obstruction | |
|   In the newborn | 1–5 % |
|   In > newborns | 0.1–1 % |
| Laparotomy[a] (bowel injury or adhesion-related strangulation or ischemia as for the newborn) | 1–5 % |
| *Rare significant/serious problems* | |
| Infection[a] | 0.1–1 % |
| Neural injury[a] | |
|   Ilioinguinal nerve | 0.1–1 % |
|   Iliohypogastric nerve | 0.1–1 % |
| Vascular injury – artery or vein | 0.1–1 % |
| Spermatic cord injury[a] (parts of vas have been found in 0.5 % of operative specimens of the sac) | 0.1–1 % |
| *Less serious complications* | |
| Pain/discomfort/tenderness(<2 months; usually only days)[a] | 5–20 % |
| Pain/discomfort/tenderness(>2 months) | 0.1–1 % |
| Scrotal/labial swelling | 5–20 % |
| Urinary retention | 0.1–1 % |
| Dehiscence[a] (rare, may occur after testicular infarction) | <0.1 % |
| Dimpling/deformity of the skin[a] | 0.1–1 % |
| Wound scarring (all) | 0.1–1 % |
| Drain tube(s)[a] | 0.1–1 % |

[a]Dependent on underlying pathology, anatomy, surgical technique, and preferences

index repair was on the right. Gonadal infarction and injury is usually a consequence of the problem, rather than a surgical complication per se, but is important to discuss preoperatively where practicable.

**Major Complications**

The **loss of the gonad** from venous infarction or torsion is a serious consequence. **Bowel injury** is rare in children, but can be significant especially after bowel incarceration, obstruction, or infarction with perforation. In the neonate, an appendix in the hernia can cause problems with deep-seated and systemic infection (and the rare T-antigen exposure) if the appendix has infarcted in the hernia, which cannot be predicted preoperatively. **Infection** also increases the risk of **dehiscence**, especially if nonabsorbable sutures are used.

---

**Consent and Risk Reduction**

**Main Points to Explain**

- GA risk
- Pain/discomfort
- Bleeding/hematoma*
- Infection (local/systemic)*
- Urinary obstruction*
- Risk of other abdominal organ injury*
- Gonad loss
- Hernia recurrence*
- Risks without surgery*

  **\*Dependent on pathology, comorbidities, and surgery performed**

---

## Surgery for Exomphalos (Omphalocele)

### Description

Exomphalos (also termed omphalocele) is an abdominal wall defect that is nearly always picked up by antenatal ultrasound, if one has been done. Exomphalos occurs in approximately 1: 5,000–6,000 live births. There is a field defect in the abdominal wall, which may be small – "exomphalos minor" – or may be large and remain within the abdominal area – "exomphalos major" (which is large enough to contain liver). One subgroup, the "giant exomphalos," has a lesion bigger than the head, the lungs are hypoplastic, and the mortality is high. An even more massive defect is where the lesion extends up into the chest – the "thoracoabdominal cleft." As the exomphalos with its field defect extends further and further, so more and more structures are involved, and the mortality rises. With thoracoabdominal cleft, for example, when picked up antenatally, most fetuses will die before birth, and those that are live-born will have a high mortality.

In a large exomphalos, there is a broad-based midline defect that can extend extensively up and down the abdomen, thorax, or pelvis, with defects in the organs within that field. The lesion is covered by a membrane that is probably the remnant of the ectoderm and the endoderm, where the muscle somites did not grow between these two layers. Severe versions in the lower abdomen are often associated with exstrophy of the urinary bladder; severe lesions in the upper abdomen and thorax are associated with exstrophy of the heart, heart defects, midline chest wall defects, and underdeveloped lungs. There may be associated lethal chromosome defects, but these are surprisingly more often associated with the smaller exomphalos minor.

The closure of a major exomphalos (one containing most of the liver) or giant exomphalos (where the lesion is bigger than the baby's head) can be very difficult. Where the exomphalos is large, a staged procedure is often used to gradually force the viscera back into the abnormally small abdomen over a period of 7–10 days. The covering membrane is usually removed at birth to be replaced with a tough Silastic sheet or polyvinyl bag (the silo), which in turn is used to force the viscera back into the abdomen as fast as can be tolerated. Usually a muscle or fascial sheath (using flaps of rectus sheath turned medially) can be achieved, but for giant exomphalos, the procedure may have to be staged over years after initial primary skin closure alone. The mortality can be high, especially with large, repeated, or complicated procedures.

**Anatomical Points**

For omphalocele (exomphalos) additional defects are present in up to 70 % of patients (higher when detected in utero, as the most complex cases die in utero). The size of the defect determines the anatomical disturbance necessitating surgical correction. The extent of herniation and amount of abdominal wall available for reconstruction can vary considerably with the degree of the field defect involved. Accordingly, the surgery has to be individualized. For thoracoabdominal clefts, the heart defects, the pericardial defect, the diaphragmatic defects, and pulmonary hypoplasia increase risks and may make surgery almost impossible.

**Perspective**

See Table 3.2. Exomphalos, in its various forms, has complications proportional to the amount of anatomical disturbance and associated organ defects. The early complications of abdominal wall repair are mainly related to respiratory insufficiency, either due to the force used to reduce the viscera or due to primary pulmonary hypoplasia or both. Infection can be problematic when the defect cannot be closed quickly, especially where the closure is not ideal. Silastic may be used as a device to force the contents in, as a temporary device to get the abdomen closed placed beneath the skin, but it commonly becomes infected. Staged repairs are used and collagen matrix "Surgi-sis®" is getting some usage to leave a stronger scar where the muscles cannot be brought together for exomphalos. Absorbable materials are preferred for closure where possible, and nonabsorbable patch materials are usually avoided. For patients in multi-organ failure, skin closure with later definitive surgery is often used. Nonabsorbable patches nearly always become infected and nonabsorbable sutures may cause suture erosion where there has been difficult closure. Even "PDS®" (polydioxanone suture) may last too long and cause problems. There are often small incisional herniae especially where there has been a flapped fascial repair. Where the muscles cannot be brought together at the first session, then a large ventral hernia has to be dealt with as a later staged repair. Even if the muscles can be brought together, they often drift apart again leaving a low-profile dome of scar tissue with the centrally placed liver lying directly underneath this. Inability to close the abdominal wall with tearing of the Silastic sac from the abdominal wall

**Table 3.2** Surgery for exomphalos (omphalocele) estimated frequency of complications, risks, and consequences

| Complications, risks, and consequences | Estimated frequency |
| --- | --- |
| *Most significant/serious complications* | |
| Infection (higher with more severe defects)[a] | 20–50 % |
| Bleeding or hematoma formation[a] | 5–20 % |
| Numbness/altered sensation | 1–5 % |
| Hernia recurrence[a] (10 year) | 1–5 % |
| Cardiorespiratory failure (especially high with congenital heart disease)[a] | 5–20 % |
| Multisystem organ failure (especially high with congenital heart disease)[a] | 5–20 % |
| Prolonged ventilation[a] | >80 % |
| TPN (total parenteral nutrition)[a] | 50–80 % |
| Suture abscess +/− suture sinus[a] | 1–5 % |
| Small bowel obstruction (later) | 20–50 % |
| Dehiscence[a] | 20–50 % |
| Death[a] | 20–50 % |
| *Less serious complications* | |
| Pain/discomfort/tenderness(<2 months) | 20–50 % |
| Pain/discomfort/tenderness(>2 months) | 0.1–1 % |
| Seroma formation | 5–20 % |
| Scarring/dimpling/deformity of the skin[a] | >80 % |
| Drain tube(s)[a] | 50–80 % |

[a]Dependent on underlying pathology, disease extent, anatomy, surgical technique, and preferences

muscles can occur, causing subsequent increased difficulty in later surgery, with sepsis and multi-organ failure. Most babies have to be ventilated for a prolonged period postoperatively and especially where the viscera are being forced back in. Total parenteral nutrition (TPN) is often required, with its associated metabolic and septic complications. Death occurs in about 30 % of live-born babies with a giant exomphalos, and in utero mortality occurs in about 50 % of complex patients detected on antenatal ultrasound, that is, death occurs before or at birth.

## Major Complications

**Death,** early and late **bowel obstruction, failure to close the defect, respiratory insufficiency, and ureteric obstruction** can arise from the pressure being used. **Infection** may be a problem, with skin organisms predominating, unless bowel injury has occurred. The presence of a major foreign body (the silo) may cause infection where it is sutured to the muscle and can contaminate the bowel in the silo. Nonabsorbable sutures can increase bacterial colonization and the risk of infection. **Bleeding** is seldom severe unless an omental or organ injury occurs. **Portosystemic anastomoses** around the umbilicus can produce annoying bleeding, but is rarely severe. **Hernia recurrence** rates for these herniae are rather high and further increased in the presence of extensive abdominal wall deficiencies and infection.

When an exomphalos major is being forced back, then **abdominal compartment syndromes** can arise from high pressures. If the liver is being forced more than the rest of the viscera, then **liver infarction** can occur, especially in those with anatomical anomalies of the blood supply. Where the pressure is more severe below the liver, the **ureteric obstruction** can arise causing postrenal failure. Obviously the pressure being utilized has to be tailored to achieve reduction, while avoiding these major issues. **Death** is a serious risk without surgery, but postoperative **multisystem organ failure** and **sepsis** remain major determinants of mortality.

---

**Consent and Risk Reduction**

**Main Points to Explain**

- GA risk
- Pain/discomfort
- Bleeding/hematoma*
- Infection (local/systemic)*
- Urinary obstruction*
- Risk of organ ischemia/infarction
- Risk of other abdominal organ injury*
- Possible further surgery*
- Hernia recurrence
- Risks without surgery*
- Death*

**\*Dependent on pathology, comorbidities, and surgery performed**

---

## Surgery for Gastroschisis

### Description

Gastroschisis is a condition that is a mechanical accident where the midgut loop ruptures out through the side of an apparently normal umbilical cord with a normal abdominal wall. This leads to protrusion of small bowel and occasionally other viscera into the amniotic cavity, from the base of the umbilical cord. The defect is becoming much more common and appears to be a vascular accident, where the frequency has been shown to increase in young mothers taking vasoactive drugs, such as cocaine. The incidence of gastroschisis in the general female reproductive age range is about 1 per 5,000 live births, but 1 per 200 live births in pregnant women under 18 years of age.

Because the intestine is protruding, irritated by amniotic fluid, it is thick walled, edematous, and shortened. As a result, there is a prolonged period of bowel dysmotility after birth that can last for life. Sections of the gut can lie over the sharp edge of the small defect and can infarct in utero. Short bowel syndrome may then occur so that 5–10 % may die or require a small bowel transplant. Up to 70 % of gastroschisis patients can have the herniated viscera returned to the abdomen primarily without the use of polyvinyl bag "silos" as the abdominal wall has its normal potential.

## Anatomical Points

The size of the defect can vary, as can the site, degree and length of bowel affected. Anatomical variants causing vascular or bowel obstruction may complicate the surgical anatomy and dictate resection of small bowel or more complex repairs, with attendant associated complications.

## Perspective

See Table 3.3. Gastroschisis is not usually associated with pulmonary hypoplasia, so lung problems are less frequent overall. The abdominal cavity is fully developed, but tends to be small because the gut has not been present inside to expand it, as the body grows. Even staged closure is relatively easy in comparison to exomphalos. Gastroschisis is a problem especially for young mothers. They require a great deal of care to get the child growing properly, and nearly all have problems with constipation because of the motility problems. Those with short bowel are often hospitalized frequently and for months, with or without transplantation. The abdominal wall repair can be associated with respiratory insufficiency, primarily due to the tightness when the viscera are reduced. Infection can occur from cutaneous or bowel organisms, especially when bowel injury occurs in utero or at surgery. Abdominal prosthetic patches are rarely required, and absorbable sutures are typically preferred.

## Major Complications

**Infection** may be a problem, with skin organisms predominating unless bowel injury has occurred. Since foreign material is seldom used, infection rates are generally lower than for exomphalos repairs. Nonabsorbable sutures can increase bacterial colonization and the risk of infection. **Bleeding** is seldom severe unless an omental, bowel, or organ injury occurs. **Hernia recurrence** rates for these herniae are moderate and further increased in the presence of infection, poor healing, multisystem organ failure, or nutritional deficiency. Lifelong immunosuppressants following SB transplantation or home **chronic TPN** may be necessary if short bowel syndrome occurs. **Liver failure** may ensue. Overall, **multisystem organ failure** and **death** are not common. **Nutritional deficiency**, **short bowel syndrome,** and **bowel dysmotility** can be significant chronic problems. Repeated or **prolonged hospitalization** can be a significant consequence.

**Table 3.3** Surgery for gastroschisis estimated frequency of complications, risks, and consequences

| Complications, risks, and consequences | Estimated frequency |
|---|---|
| *Most significant/serious complications* | |
| Infection (higher with more severe defects) | 20–50 % |
| Bleeding or hematoma formation[a] | 5–20 % |
| Numbness/altered sensation | 1–5 % |
| Hernia recurrence[a] (10 year) | 1–5 % |
| Cardiorespiratory failure (especially high with congenital heart disease)[a] | 5–20 % |
| Multisystem organ failure (especially high with congenital heart disease)[a] | 5–20 % |
| Prolonged ventilation[a] | 50–80 % |
| TPN (total parenteral nutrition)[a] | 50–80 % |
| Bowel dysmotility[a] | >80 % |
| Malabsorption and failure to thrive[a] | 5–20 % |
| Suture abscess +/– suture sinus[a] | 1–5 % |
| Small bowel obstruction (later) or pseudo-obstruction for life[a] | 20–50 % |
| Multiple hospital admissions (for all complications)[a] | 20–50 % |
| Liver failure (often from short bowel syndrome and TPN)[a] | 5–20 % |
| Small bowel transplant[a] | 5–20 % |
| Dehiscence[a] | 20–50 % |
| Death[a] | 5–20 % |
| *Less serious complications* | |
| Pain/discomfort/tenderness(<2 months) | 20–50 % |
| Pain/discomfort/tenderness(>2 months) | 0.1–1 % |
| Seroma formation | 5–20 % |
| Scarring/dimpling/deformity of the skin[a] | 1–5 % |
| Drain tube(s)[a] | 1–5 % |

[a]Dependent on underlying pathology, anatomy, surgical technique, and preferences

**Consent and Risk Reduction**

**Main Points to Explain**

- GA risk
- Pain/discomfort
- Bleeding/hematoma*
- Infection (local/systemic)*
- Nutritional deficiency
- Risk of other abdominal organ injury*
- Hernia recurrence
- Possible further surgery*
- Risks without surgery*
- Death*

**\*Dependent on pathology, comorbidities, and surgery performed**

## General Abdominal Surgery

### Open Pyloromyotomy for Pyloric Stenosis

#### Description

General anesthesia is used. Pyloric stenosis is hypertrophy of the pyloric muscle and occurs in approximately 1:200 male and about 1:1,000 female live births (i.e., 85 % are male). It typically develops in the first 4–6 weeks of life in the first-born male. The aim is to divide the constricting hypertrophic muscle that encircles the pyloric region, using a longitudinal (Ramstedt) pyloromyotomy, exposing the underlying intact mucosa. The pyloromyotomy allows drainage by incising longitudinally, approximately 1–2 cm, through the muscle wall of the pyloric canal from immediately proximal to the duodenal bulb and then back to the antrum. This longitudinal incision deliberately leaves the muscle wall gaping, down to the intact mucosa, which then balloons into the muscle defect allowing passive drainage of gastric contents.

#### Anatomical Points

The anatomy of the pylorus is relatively constant; however, the extent of the pyloric hypertrophy may vary, proximally up the antral wall. The hypertrophy always ends abruptly at the junction of the pylorus and duodenum, with no duodenal extension, and there is a normal duodenal bulb. The degree of preoperative obstruction, projectile vomiting, and consequent acid-base and electrolyte imbalance will vary considerably and has to be corrected prior to surgery.

#### Perspective

See Table 3.4. Most of the complications are of a minor nature, and children usually recover rapidly from surgery. Major complications are related to perforation of the mucosa, wound infection, recurrence of pyloric obstruction, and rarely later complications of small bowel obstruction. Correction of preoperative electrolyte disturbances and ensuring adequate nutrition are important considerations.

#### Major Complications

Inadvertent **perforation** and **leakage** may be serious and occasionally not recognized at operation, leading to **intra-abdominal infection** and **abscess** formation. If the perforation is recognized and closed during operation, the risk of infection is approximately doubled, but if not recognized, then intra-abdominal sepsis is almost inevitable. **Infection and multisystem failure** may be catastrophic, although **death**

**Table 3.4** Open pyloromyotomy for pyloric stenosis estimated frequency of complications, risks, and consequences

| Complications, risks, and consequences | Estimated frequency |
| --- | --- |
| *Most significant/serious complications* | |
| Infection[a] | |
|   Subcutaneous/wound | 5–20 % |
|   Intra-abdominal | 0.1–1 % |
|   Systemic | 0.1–1 % |
| Bleeding or hematoma formation[a] | 1–5 % |
| Wound breakdown and evisceration | 5–20 % |
| Perforation of the mucosa or duodenum | 5–20 % |
| Reflux esophagitis | 5–20 % |
| Delayed gastric emptying[a] | 20–50 % |
| Recurrence/persistence of pyloric obstruction[a] | 1–5 % |
| Mortality[a] | 0.1–1 % |
| Mortality <u>without</u> surgery | 20–50 % |
| *Rare significant/serious problems* | |
| Liver injury[a] | 0.1–1 % |
| Small bowel obstruction (early or late; lifetime)[a] [Adhesion formation] | 0.1–1 % |
| Subphrenic abscess | <0.1 % |
| Multisystem failure (renal, pulmonary, cardiac failure) | <0.1 % |
| *Less serious complications* | |
| Paralytic ileus | 1–5 % |
| Slow recovery requiring prolonged feeding with small frequent feeds | 5–20 % |
| Wound scarring (poor cosmesis/wound deformity) | 1–5 % |
| Incisional hernia | 5–20 % |
| Prolonged use of nasogastric tube[a] | 1–5 % |

[a]Dependent on underlying pathology, anatomy, surgical technique, and preferences

is very rare. **Bleeding** is rare and is usually controlled at surgery. **Wound infection** is common and occurs especially in malnourished infants with severe prolonged vomiting prior to presentation and diagnosis. **Wound dehiscence** and consequent **hernia formation** may result. **Persistent pyloric stenosis** can result from inadequate division of the hypertrophic muscle, but true **recurrent pyloric stenosis** is very rare. **Small bowel obstruction** is rare but may occur from postoperative adhesions, even many years later.

**Consent and Risk Reduction**

**Main Points to Explain**

- GA risk
- Pain/discomfort
- Bleeding/hematoma*
- Infection (local/systemic)*

- Risk of other abdominal organ injury*
- Perforation*
- Recurrence of stenosis
- Possible further surgery*
- Risks without surgery*

   **\*Dependent on pathology, comorbidities, and surgery performed**

## Laparoscopic Pyloromyotomy for Pyloric Stenosis

### Description

General anesthesia is used. Pyloric stenosis is hypertrophy of the pyloric muscle and occurs in approximately 1:200 male and about 1:1,000 female live births (i.e., 85 % are male). It typically develops in the first 4–6 weeks of life in the first-born male. The aim is to divide the constricting hypertrophic muscle that encircles the pyloric region, using a longitudinal (Ramstedt) pyloromyotomy, exposing the underlying imperforated mucosa. The pyloromyotomy allows drainage by incising longitudinally, approximately 1–2 cm, through the muscle wall of the pyloric canal from immediately proximal to the duodenal bulb and then back to the antrum. This longitudinal incision deliberately leaves the muscle wall gaping, down to the intact mucosa, which then balloons into the muscle defect allowing passive drainage of gastric contents. Approximately half of all pyloromyotomies are now carried out laparoscopically even in premature babies. This frequency will continue to increase, as it is a good training procedure for younger surgeons starting laparoscopy in pediatric patients. In all babies (down to 1.0 Kg), there is no need for access ports other than for the 3 mm telescope. The other 3 mm instruments are placed directly through small stab wounds so that the cosmetic results are superior.

### Anatomical Points

The anatomy of the pylorus is relatively constant; however, the extent of the pyloric hypertrophy may vary, proximally up the antral wall. The hypertrophy always ends abruptly at the junction of the pylorus and duodenum, with no duodenal extension, and there is a normal duodenal bulb. The degree of preoperative obstruction, projectile vomiting, and consequent acid-base and electrolyte imbalance will vary considerably and has to be corrected prior to surgery. Adhesions from previous surgery or an enlarged liver may make laparoscopic access more difficult.

### Perspective

See Table 3.5. Most of the complications are of a minor nature, and children usually recover rapidly from surgery. With laparoscopic approaches, the risk of wound

**Table 3.5** Laparoscopic pyloromyotomy for pyloric stenosis estimated frequency of complications, risks, and consequences

| Complications, risks, and consequences | Estimated frequency |
|---|---|
| *Most significant/serious complications* | |
| Infection[a] | |
|   Subcutaneous/wound | 5–20 % |
|   Intra-abdominal | 0.1–1 % |
|   Systemic | 0.1–1 % |
| Bleeding or hematoma formation[a] | 1–5 % |
| Wound breakdown and evisceration | 5–20 % |
| Perforation of the mucosa or duodenum | 5–20 % |
| Reflux esophagitis | 5–20 % |
| Delayed gastric emptying | 20–50 % |
| Conversion to open operation | 1–5 % |
| Recurrence/persistence of pyloric obstruction | 1–5 % |
| Mortality <u>without</u> surgery | 20–50 % |
| *Rare significant/serious problems* | |
| Pneumothorax | 0.1–1 % |
| Gas embolus | 0.1–1 % |
| Liver injury | 0.1–1 % |
| Small bowel obstruction (early or late; lifetime)[a] [Adhesion formation] | 0.1–1 % |
| Subphrenic abscess | <0.1 % |
| Multisystem failure (renal, pulmonary, cardiac failure) | <0.1 % |
| Mortality | 0.1–1 % |
| *Less serious complications* | |
| Paralytic ileus | 1–5 % |
| Slow recovery requiring prolonged feeding with small frequent feeds | 5–20 % |
| Surgical emphysema | 1–5 % |
| Pain/tenderness | |
|   Acute (<4 weeks) | 5–20 % |
|   Chronic (>4 weeks) | <0.1 % |
| Port-site herniae | 5–20 % |
| Wound scarring (poor cosmesis/wound deformity) | 1–5 % |
| Incisional hernia | 5–20 % |
| Prolonged use of nasogastric tube[a] | 1–5 % |

[a]Dependent on underlying pathology, anatomy, surgical technique, and preferences

infection, wound dehiscence, and incisional hernia is reduced. Major complications are related to perforation of the mucosa, wound infection, recurrence of pyloric obstruction, and rarely later complications of small bowel obstruction. Correction of preoperative electrolyte disturbances and ensuring adequate nutrition are important considerations. With laparoscopy, there is an increased risk of mucosal perforation in the pyloric canal and of tears to the duodenal cap as the grasper holds the duodenum during division and spreading of the very mobile, hypertrophied pylorus muscle. Laparoscopic entry is associated with the complication of herniation of the omentum, or rarely bowel, through any of the port-site wounds, of about 5–10 %.

**Major Complications**

Inadvertent **perforation** and **leakage** may be serious and occasionally not recognized at operation, leading to **intra-abdominal infection** and **abscess** formation. If the perforation is recognized and closed during operation, the risk of infection is approximately doubled, but if not recognized, then intra-abdominal sepsis is almost inevitable. **Infection and multisystem failure** may be catastrophic, although **death** is very rare. **Bleeding** is rare and is usually controlled at surgery. **Wound infection** is common and occurs especially in malnourished infants with severe prolonged vomiting prior to presentation and diagnosis. **Wound dehiscence** and consequent **hernia formation** may result. **Persistent pyloric stenosis** can result from inadequate division of the hypertrophic muscle, but true **recurrent pyloric stenosis** is very rare. **Small bowel obstruction** is rare but may occur from postoperative adhesions, even many years later. **Gas embolus** and **major vascular injury** are additional serious, although very rare, complications of the laparoscopic approach. **Conversion to open operation** is a small but significant risk rather than a complication per se.

**Consent and Risk Reduction**

**Main Points to Explain**

- GA risk
- Pain/discomfort
- Bleeding/hematoma*
- Infection (local/systemic)*
- Risk of other abdominal organ injury*
- Perforation*
- Recurrence of stenosis
- Possible further surgery*
- Risks without surgery*

   *Dependent on pathology, comorbidities, and surgery performed

# Congenital Diaphragmatic Hernia Repair

### Description

General anesthesia is used. Congenital diaphragmatic hernia is a defect in the diaphragm that occurs before birth, leaving a free communication between the chest and abdominal cavities. The most common form is a posterolateral defect through the foramen of Bochdalek and occurs on the left side in over ¾ of cases. Abdominal contents in the chest often inhibit lung development and growth. After birth, this lack of lung volume and maturation makes gas exchange difficult or impossible.

Even if the baby survives the immediate period after birth, higher than normal pulmonary vascular resistance promotes persistence of the right to left ductal and cardiac shunting of blood through a ductus arteriosus and patent foramen ovale (persistence of fetal circulation). The size of the defect and degree of herniation of contents are directly associated with the risk of complications and mortality. Larger-sized defects are less likely to close. The larger the defect, the more medially it extends until the liver herniates upward through a large hole with medial extension. If the liver has rotated up into the chest, then the baby is more likely to die than if the liver is in the abdomen. CDH is often associated with many other abnormalities: cardiac and chromosomal which often prove to be lethal. The mortality is probably 30–50 % for those detected antenatally (as long as there is no other lethal defect – the isolated CDH), but for those seen to have liver in the chest on antenatal ultrasound, the mortality is greater than 90 %.

Emergency surgery is no longer the treatment of choice. The patient must be stabilized prior to surgery, and this may take days or even weeks. When there is sufficient respiratory reserve for the patient to be able to tolerate the surgery, then a transverse upper abdominal incision is used. In those that have a good prognosis, closure of the defect is usually straightforward as the defect will not be big, and there will usually be good muscle shelves that can be unfolded. If the defect is large or the diaphragm is completely absent, then partial closure can be obtained as above, and the rest (or the whole diaphragm) can be closed using an abdominal wall flap or Gerota's fascia (the perirenal fascia is dissected up from the lower pole of the kidney to the top, leaving the attachment to the upper pole of the kidney as a hinge from the kidney which has become more popular recently). Using a muscle flap leaves a weakness in the abdominal wall that produces a permanent bulge and possibly scoliosis later in life as the child grows. Use of Gerota's fascia has only been introduced recently, but appears to be an effective closure without such side effects. Closing the defect with synthetic material has been used in the past, but this material does not grow with the child so that there is a very high rate of recurrence as the attachments give way. Suturing the anterior ribs to the posterior ribs at the lateral end of the defect can be used, but may lead to severe chest wall deformity and a small volume stomach later, as there is no space between the ribs for the stomach to act as a reservoir.

**Anatomical Points**

The diaphragm is formed from the pleuroperitoneal membranes, the septum transversum, the dorsal mesentery of the esophagus, and the body wall. The closure of the pleuroperitoneal canals joining the thorax and abdomen starts to occur by about the 6th week of gestation and should be complete by approximately 10 weeks of gestation. Failure to close fully leads to persistence of the posterolateral pleuroperitoneal canal – the foramen of Bochdalek – which occurs in approximately 1:2,200 conceptions and 1:4,000 live births, as many die before birth of multiple anomalies. Some 80 % occur on the left side. Herniation through the retrosternal area – foramen of Morgagni – is a rare defect.

**Perspective**

See Table 3.6. Death occurs in approximately 50 % of cases when CDH is discovered antenatally and higher in preterm infants. The time at which the defect stops closing determines the outcome. If the defect stops closing early in gestation, the liver rotates into the chest, and being more solid than intestine causes more damage. The abdominal viscera (liver and intestine) push the left lung up and the heart over to the right and compress the right lung as well. So both lungs are compressed. As a result both lungs are small but also undergo a maturation arrest. The larger the defect, the more immature and small the lungs and the more complex the surgery to close it effectively. The presence of additional anomalies also contributes to the mortality and complications. Delayed lung maturation leads to a lung histology that is similar to the lung development of a very preterm baby. In addition, the lungs are smaller, so the clinician has to support a full-term baby with lungs that are far too small, and have arrested development (in the pseudoglandular phase) so that ventilator-induced chronic lung disease (of the newborn) frequently occurs, but usually resolves by a year of age – in survivors. This may be responsible for late deaths weeks and months after birth. Viral infections during this period may well tip the baby into respiratory failure and death. Coexistence of cardiac anomalies increases the mortality. The neonate is typically completely unaware of this as he/she will be paralyzed, ventilated, and sedated. When CDH is detected later (up to 20 years after birth), then pain and awareness are often more of an issue.

**Major Complications**

**Death** occurs in up to 50 % of those born alive, and death has already occurred in another 20 % before birth or immediately after birth due to the basic inability to ventilate these babies. If the liver was seen to be in the chest before birth, and if the lung to head ratio is less than 0.8 on antenatal ultrasound, death before, during, or after birth is likely in more than 90 % of fetuses. In those that survive the immediate period after birth, the next major hurdle is the **high pulmonary vascular resistance**, which maintains a "persistent fetal circulation". There is often a supra-systemic pulmonary blood pressure, so that blood shunts away from the lungs at the level of the ductus arteriosus and the foramen ovale. Because of the high pressure, the right side of the heart also fails. Support therefore becomes complex, often involving pulmonary vasodilators such as inhaled nitric oxide, longer-term sildenafil therapy, and right ventricular support. Long before this occurs, the baby is often placed on oscillating **ventilation** to try to reduce lung damage, but long-term data has not shown any improvement in survival for those that are oscillated. This situation of hypoxia, shunting, and cardiac failure (leading to multi-organ failure) has a high mortality and is exceptionally difficult to treat. Secondary **lung infection** is not uncommon and may affect either lung. Viral pneumonitis is common months after the surgery, and in those that have only just survived the initial problems, the infection may well tip the baby into terminal respiratory failure. If the fluid in the almost empty left hemithorax becomes infected, this rapidly leads to generalized sepsis and multi-organ failure. Overventilation leading to **pneumothorax** or **persistent air leak** creates a situation that cannot be resolved on conventional ventilation.

**Table 3.6** Surgery for congenital diaphragmatic hernia estimated frequency of complications, risks, and consequences

| Complications, risks, and consequences | Estimated frequency |
|---|---|
| ***Most significant/serious complications*** | |
| Infection | |
|    Subcutaneous/wound | 1–5 % |
|    Intrathoracic (pneumonia; pleural) | 1–5 % |
|    Mediastinitis | 0.1–1 % |
|    Systemic | 0.1–1 % |
| Prolonged assisted ventilation[a,b] | 80 % |
| Gastroesophageal reflux | 50–80 % |
| Chronic lung disease; pulmonary failure[a] | 50–80 % |
| Diaphragmatic injury/dysfunction/paresis | 5–20 % |
| Small bowel obstruction | 5–20 % |
| Scoliosis and chest wall deformities (postoperative)[a] (especially where prosthetic patches or muscle flaps have been used) | 5–20 % |
| Volvulus | 1–5 % |
| Multisystem organ failure (renal, pulmonary, cardiac failure)[a] (ultimate cause of death in approximately 50 % of neonates) | 20–50 % |
| Mortality | |
|    Term infants[a] | 20–50 % |
|    Preterm infants[a] (includes those detected antenatally – usual today) | 50–80 % |
| Mortality <u>without</u> surgery (almost 100 % for severe early defects)[a] | >80 % |
| ***Rare significant/serious problems*** | |
| Bleeding/hematoma formation | |
|    Wound | 0.1–1 % |
|    Hemothorax | 0.1–1 % |
|    Pulmonary contusion | 0.1–1 % |
| Surgical emphysema | 0.1–1 % |
| Persistent air leak[a] | 0.1–1 % |
| Deep venous thrombosis | 0.1–1 % |
| Osteomyelitis of ribs[a] | <0.1 % |
| ***Less serious complications*** | |
| Pain/tenderness[a,b] | |
|    Acute (<4weeks) | 5–20 % |
|    Chronic (>4 weeks) | <0.1 % |
| Wound scarring | 5–20 % |
| Deformity of rib/chest or skin (poor cosmesis) | 1–5 % |

[a]Note: Dependent on the extent and underlying disease/pathology, location of disease, and/or surgical preference which will alter the relative risks
[b]The neonate will usually be completely unaware being paralyzed, ventilated, and sedated; for repairs in later life, it can be a problem

Oscillation or ECMO may have to be used to retrieve this situation. ECMO as a primary treatment for CDH to get the neonate through the first few days or weeks of life has not achieved universal acceptance and is rarely used in Australia. ECMO as a retrieval from an air leak can be effective.

There is an emerging group of neonates that now only just survive, as we get gradually better at retrieving the hypoxic shunting baby. These babies are now managed with permissive hypercapnea and apparently less than ideal hypoventilation (which drastically reduces lung damage and mimics the levels of tissue oxygenation that was present before birth). These babies have previously rarely seen problems.

Moderate to severe **tracheobronchomalacia,** where major airway collapse can occur from the soft walls of the airways, from the larynx to the major bronchi can occur. To take these patients off a ventilator, a **tracheostomy** may be required for months until the trachea and bronchi become more rigid and are able to support themselves. This will take months or up to a year. Another problem is **persisting pulmonary hypertension** that may go on for months. In the past this was an acute problem only, as the patient either recovered or died. Now, the patients are surviving through the acute phase (weeks) only for the problem to persist for months, if not a year or so.

**Multisystem organ failure** is extremely serious and is the usual mode of death in those that survive long enough to be ventilated. This is usually the result of the inability to oxygenate the patient or generalized sepsis. Cardiac anomalies will contribute to multi-organ failure, so that the ultimate cause of death in these patients is often a combination of problems leading to this scenario. Once established, there is a high mortality. **Mortality** is greater for infants with large herniae, those with a large volume of liver in the chest, cardiac disease, bilateral herniae, and in very preterm/low-birth-weight infants (<1,500 g). Those with chromosomal anomalies, e.g., trisomy 13 or 18, rarely survive birth and often die in utero. Even if they survive birth, they soon die, and treatment would not be a viable option.

<u>For repeat surgery</u>: In the neonate, **bowel perforation** is rare, but may occur in repeat surgery especially where a prosthetic patch has been used, has torn off its attachments as the baby grows, and then has to be dissected off the colon. Then the subsequent leakage and infection may be devastating. Pleural space infection (**empyema**) may follow leakage from the bowel, but is virtually unheard of in the first operation.

---

**Consent and Risk Reduction**

**Main Points to Explain**

- GA risk
- Pain/discomfort
- Bleeding/hematoma*
- Infection (local/systemic)*
- Nutritional deficiency
- Risk of other abdominal organ injury*
- Hernia recurrence
- Persistent pneumothorax
- Possible further surgery*
- Risks without surgery*
- Multisystem organ failure
- Death*

**\*Dependent on pathology, comorbidities, and surgery performed**

# Biliary Atresia and Choledochal Cyst Surgery: Biliary Bypass Drainage: Roux-en-Y Hepaticojejunostomy (The Kasai Procedure)

## Description

The aim is to restore bile flow from the liver to the intestine by resecting, bypassing, or relieving the obstruction.

**Biliary atresia** occurs in about 1 in 10,000 live births (and may be higher in Asian populations), resulting in fibrous obliteration of the biliary tree (may occur early in life probably as a form of neonatal sclerosing cholangitis).

**Choledochal cysts** are at least fivefold (1:50,000) less common (but also relatively higher in Asians and females) and comprise a group of congenital dilatations of the bile ducts. The most common in the neonate is a "fusiform" dilation of the common bile duct and common hepatic duct up to the confluence of the left and right hepatic ducts. In the neonate, choledochal cysts may show some of the features of biliary atresia, and the two can coexist. For example, it is not uncommon to see a choledochal cyst in the CBD, accompanied with classical histological biliary atresia in the more distal CBD.

Long-term cholangiocarcinomas may develop in unresected choledochal cysts, a few before age 25. But, only 57 % of the cholangiocarcinomas occur in the area of the cyst. Therefore, nearly 50 % will occur in the residual biliary system after the cyst is removed and bypassed. This implies that the whole of the biliary tree is at risk. Surgery depends on the type of abnormality and extent of obstruction. For the more common choledochal cysts in childhood, the choice is limited to (i) a Roux-en-Y jejunostomy anastomosed to the common hepatic duct or (difficult in a neonate) to the right and left hepatic ducts after "fish-mouthing" the inferior borders of those ducts or (ii) a cholecocho-duodenostomy, where the common hepatic duct is joined to the upper border of the duodenum. The latter can be done quite effectively laparoscopically in the child. Close follow-up is usually required to detect late stenosis, which may produce multiple stones within the biliary tree above the stenosis; or in the case of choledochal cysts, cholangiocarcinoma of the remaining bile duct(s) can occur. Occasionally, resection of the short, affected portion of extrahepatic bile duct can be performed with primary end-end anastomosis.

In *biliary atresia*, the Kasai portoenterostomy joins the porta hepatis to a Roux-en-Y jejunal loop, after removing the scar tissue at the hepatic plate, leaving only the inner layers of the plate, so as to avoid entering the liver parenchyma. The dissection is carried out as far laterally as possible, and the lymphatics are preserved (not coagulated) as they may be the source of future bile drainage. In biliary atresia, one third of patients will never drain bile and go into liver failure within months of birth. Of the two thirds that drain bile, only half of them (one third or those operated on) will continue to drain bile beyond 5 years of age and may reach 20–30 years of age before they require transplant.

## Anatomical Points

Knowledge of the common and uncommon biliary and vascular anatomical variants is essential for reducing mishap during biliary surgery. For choledochal cyst, the cyst is dissected out by peeling it away from its surrounding tissues, bearing in mind the anatomical variants that can occur. For biliary atresia, scar tissue is present, so the fibrous band that represents the GB is dissected down to the "fibrous pyramid" that represents the CHD and the right and left hepatic ducts, and then the vessels are identified one by one around this pyramid, taking care to identify the small arteries in the neonate (and up to 3 months of age). Once that is done, the fibrous pyramid is removed down to the last inner layer of the hepatic plate. Correct identification of the common bile duct, rather than the common hepatic duct, should be confirmed to ensure that a choledochotomy is not performed in a bile duct that is too small (no luxury of choice may exist as the cyst may well go up into the CHD and even the confluence of the hepatic ducts). Even CT cholangiograms or MRCP will not usually clarify the anatomy particularly well in the very young. Preoperatively in the neonate, the choledochal cyst can occupy the whole of the abdomen, and the whole system is distorted. For the common form of choledochal cysts, the CBD, the GB and part of the CHD are involved. For intrahepatic cysts, the cyst would probably be left until the child is older, or if causing cholangitis, a liver resection (if practical with multiple cysts) may be preferable.

**Perspective**

See Table 3.7. Early major complications are related to failure to drain bile, bleeding, bile leakage, and infection, and later complications include biliary stenosis and bile duct malignancy (for cysts) and recurrent cholangitis and liver (cirrhosis) fibrosis (for those with biliary atresia (BA)). Minor complications are common and usually resolve without sequelae. Coexisting congenital disorders or anomalies, e.g., cardiac, especially left atrial isomerism, may predispose to higher risks of complications and failures. When these patterns of disease coexist with biliary atresia, they are known as syndromal forms of BA. When these syndromal forms occur, they have a far worse prognosis than the idiopathic form. Longer-term survival is dependent on disease progression, recurrent infections, cholangiocarcinoma (in choledochal cysts), and the inevitable ongoing fibrosis of the liver in biliary atresia. This leads eventually to liver failure in every patient with BA. *Liver transplantation* will typically be required for biliary atresia in the long term. So, all patients would die without transplant at some stage, 2/3 before 5 years of age. The best units internationally can obtain 40–45 % of patients out to 5 years without transplant, but if not transplanted, all eventually succumb to liver failure. Transplant can be carried out down to 5 Kg body weight and possibly less, depending on the patient, disease, and unit. Without transplant all of these patients will go into liver failure at some age and die.

For choledochal cysts, there is a high rate of stenosis and cholelithiasis usually occurring 10–20 years after the initial surgery. This may even require liver transplantation. For the Kasai procedure, death will be inevitable without liver transplant at varying times (however, the success for the Kasai procedure is only about 5 years or so of adequate drainage).

**Table 3.7** Surgery for biliary atresia and choledochal cyst estimated frequency of complications, risks, and consequences

| Complications, risks, and consequences | Estimated frequency |
|---|---|
| ***Most significant/serious complications*** | |
| Death in biliary atresia as above | |
| Late stenosis, cholelithiasis, and liver failure in choledochal cysts | |
|    Infection[a] overall | 1–5 % |
|    Subcutaneous/wound | 1–5 % |
|    Intra-abdominal/liver bed/pelvic | 0.1–1 % |
|    Liver(hepatitis; abscess) | 0.1–1 % |
|    Cholangitis | 20–50 % |
|    Systemic | 0.1–1 % |
| Bleeding/hematoma formation | |
|    Wound | 1–5 % |
|    Anastomotic; raw liver surface | 1–5 % |
|    Gastrointestinal (incl. variceal) hemorrhage | 20–50 % |
| Liver failure long term (cirrhosis)[a] | 20–50 % |
| Portal hypertension | 20–50 % |
| Bile leak/collection | 20–50 % |
| Biliary fistula[a] | 5–20 % |
| Biliary ischemia/stenosis/obstruction/cholelithiasis[a] | 20–50 % |
| Small bowel fistulae[a] | 1–5 % |
| Later cholangiocarcinoma[a] | 1–5 % |
| Mortality (10 year)[a] | 20–50 % |
| Mortality without surgery[a] | >80 % |
| ***Rare significant/serious problems*** | |
| Injury to the bowel or blood vessels | 0.1–1 % |
|    Gastric/duodenal/small bowel/colonic | |
| Bile/hepatic duct injury | 0.1–1 % |
| Liver injury | 0.1–1 % |
| Biliary ascites | 0.1–1 % |
| Failure to detect/remove calculi | 0.1–1 % |
| Jejunal fistula | 0.1–1 % |
| Small bowel ischemia | 0.1–1 % |
| Multisystem organ failure (renal, pulmonary, cardiac failure)[a] | 0.1–1 % |
| Small bowel obstruction (early or late)[a] [Anastomotic stenosis/ischemic stenosis/adhesion formation] | 0.1–1 % |
| Operative cholangiogram | |
|    Dye reaction/cholangitis/pancreatitis/radiation exposure | <0.1 % |
| Possibility of colostomy/ileostomy (very rare)[a] | 0.1–1 % |
| Pancreatitis/pancreatic injury/pancreatic cyst/pancreatic fistula[a] | 0.1–1 % |
| Aspiration pneumonitis | 0.1–1 % |
| Wound dehiscence | 0.1–1 % |
| Incisional hernia formation (delayed heavy lifting/straining) | 0.1–1 % |
| T-tube-related complications (if used) | |
| T-tube cholangiogram | |
|    Dye reaction/cholangitis/pancreatitis/radiation exposure | <0.1 % |

(continued)

**Table 3.7** (continued)

| Complications, risks, and consequences | Estimated frequency |
|---|---|
| Blockage of T-tube | 0.1–1 % |
| Dislodgment of T-tube | 1–5 % |
| Persistent biliary fistula (after removal; cholangio-cutaneous) | 0.1–1 % |
| *Less serious complications* | |
| Pain/tenderness | |
|    Acute (<4 weeks) | 5–20 % |
|    Chronic (>4 weeks) | <0.1 % |
| Seroma/lymphocele formation | 0.1–1 % |
| Muscle weakness (atrophy due to denervation esp subcostal incision) | 1–5 % |
| Paralytic ileus[a] | 50–80 % |
| Nasogastric tube[a] | 1–5 % |
| Blood transfusion | <0.1 % |
| Wound drain tube(s)[a] | 1–5 % |
| Wound scarring (poor cosmesis/wound deformity) | 1–5 % |

[a]Dependent on underlying pathology, anatomy, surgical technique, and preferences

## Major Complications

For **biliary atresia**, one of the main complications is **failure of adequate biliary drainage** and **persistent jaundice**, with continued liver fibrosis/cirrhosis no matter whether they get drainage or not. Only the relative rates change. Fibrosis is faster in those that are not drained, so that synthetic function fails earlier, with subsequent **liver cirrhosis**, also due to progressive biliary fibrosis. Paradoxically, in those that drain well, there is a higher incidence of subsequent bacterial **cholangitis**, which can be very difficult to treat, accompanied by cessation of bile drainage, and may become chronic leading to permanent loss of drainage and **liver failure**. If there is no anatomical path for drainage (e.g., failed Kasai), then there is no path for bacteria, and cholangitis does not occur. **Bile leakage** may occur and can lead to **bile ascites** or **fistula** formation, surprisingly easily controlled and usually stops within a week or two. Venous **bleeding** can be catastrophic during the procedure and difficult to control and maintain flow. **Portal hypertension** with **variceal bleeding** often occurs after a Kasai procedure and often presents a significant risk to the patient. **Cirrhosis** with fibrosis of the liver and biliary system with excretory failure is a serious problem. **Bleeding** may be severe, arising from either arterial or venous injury (more likely in the adult patient as, in the child, the arterial vessels are very small). However, bleeding usually stops, but the liver parenchyma can be devascularized, the extent of which depends on the level of injury.

For **choledochal cyst**, **biliary stricture formation** may occur at any stage postoperatively and necessitate **further surgery**. Recurrent attacks of hyperamylasemia (raised lipase also) and **pancreatitis** are not infrequent after choledochal cyst surgery and are usually mild and can be managed nonsurgically in the majority of cases. Severe pancreatitis is relatively rare. **Cholangiocarcinoma** in the remaining choledochal cyst is not uncommon, often many years later.

**Wound infection, peritonitis,** or **abscess formation** may lead to **multisystem organ failure** and **death,** but the incidence of these complications is surprisingly small for the first operation. A second exploration, after sudden cessation of bile drainage, is now rarely used and multiple operations virtually never. With repeat operations, the complication rates increase, and the complications of subsequent liver transplantation are also increased, so that repeat surgery is employed less and less. These procedures carry a significant short- and longer-term risk of further complications and **mortality**.

---

**Consent and Risk Reduction**

**Main Points to Explain**

- GA risk
- Pain/discomfort
- Bleeding/hematoma*
- Infection (local/systemic)*
- Nutritional deficiency
- Risk of other abdominal organ injury*
- Recurrent biliary stricture
- Liver failure and transplantation
- Later malignancy
- Possible further surgery*
- Risks without surgery*
- Multisystem organ failure
- Death*

*Dependent on pathology, comorbidities, and surgery performed*

---

# Surgery for Congenital Duodenal Obstruction

## Description

General anesthesia is used. Congenital duodenal obstruction is due to either duodenal atresia (75 %) or stenosis (25 %) resulting in third-trimester polyhydramnios, duodenal dilatation, and early vomiting. Duodenal atresia or stenoses due to malrotation (with Ladd's bands and/or volvulus), annular pancreas, and duodenal web represent the main underlying causes.

**Duodenal atresia** is often diagnosed antenatally. The diagnosis usually occurs late in the pregnancy so that termination is no longer possible. Approximately 30 % of those diagnosed antenatally will have a chromosomal abnormality (nearly all trisomy 21), and many duodenal atresia patients will have other abnormalities (even if they do not have a chromosomal abnormality). As a result, prenatal counseling can be complex. Duodenal atresias can present surprisingly late after birth, often after several days. The over-distended stomach empties itself immediately after birth, and the baby can then apparently tolerate small feeds for a considerable time while the stomach refills. Atresia is corrected by a duodenoduodenostomy, where the distal duodenum is rotated and flipped over the area of the obstruction to be joined to the proximal duodenum. This avoids dissecting into the area where the bile and pancreatic ducts enter the duodenum (nearly always close to the level of the obstruction).

**Duodenal stenosis** can vary, and the degree of obstruction determines the timing and severity of onset of symptoms, after birth. Occasionally, a patient with duodenal stenosis may not present for several years. The aim of surgery is either to open the obstructed area or to bypass it. A duodenal web is usually corrected by a longitudinal duodenotomy with incision or fulguration of the antimesenteric portion of the web (again to avoid damage to the bile ducts which can run either on surface of the web or usually closer to the mesenteric border). Once a web has been divided, the duodenum is closed transversely.

## Anatomical Points

The anatomy of the duodenum is determined by the type of congenital defect present and whether malrotation is also a factor. The ampulla of Vater may be injured in the surgery, largely depending on the proximity to the site of obstruction and surgery, as the bile ducts open above or below the level of obstruction, or on the actual web when present. Concurrent cardiac anomalies may cause cardiac failure postoperatively and increase mortality. Other anomalies are present frequently in association with atresia or stenosis including Down's syndrome (trisomy 21).

## Perspective

See Table 3.8. Overall mortality is often more directly related to severe associated anomalies (chromosomal and congenital) rather than the duodenal obstruction itself. Those with lethal chromosomal abnormalities (e.g., trisomy 18) may be so severe as to preclude surgery. The major surgical complication is a leak at the anastomosis. Gastric emptying will seldom be normal, and the stomach takes weeks before it is emptying adequately. This may necessitate a naso-enteric tube. Duodenal obstruction is often seen within days of birth. Intravenous feeding may be required if the stomach will not empty postoperatively. Many complications are of a minor nature, and babies recover rapidly from surgery. Major complications are related to infection, perforation, recurrence of duodenal obstruction, leakage, and later complications of small bowel obstruction. Major infections, multisystem failure, and mortality are higher in those with significant congenital anomalies, often cardiac.

**Table 3.8** Surgery for congenital duodenal obstruction estimated frequency of complications, risks, and consequences

| Complications, risks, and consequences | Estimated frequency |
|---|---|
| *Most significant/serious complications* | |
| Infection[a] | |
|   Subcutaneous/wound | 1–5 % |
|   Intra-abdominal | 5–20 % |
|   Mediastinitis | <0.1 % |
|   Systemic (especially in those with chromosomal abnormalities +/− heart disease) | 5–20 % |
| Bleeding and hematoma formation[a] | 1–5 % |
| Pancreatic injury/leakage/damage to the bile ducts | 5–20 % |
| Green bilious aspirates (universal for days or weeks after the surgery) | >80 % |
| Duodenal leak at the anastomosis | 5–20 % |
| Recurrence/persistence of duodenal obstruction (some degree of duodenal dysmotility will persist for life, so that GOR is very common) | 1–5 % |
| Reflux esophagitis (GOR) | 20–50 % |
| Multisystem failure (renal, pulmonary, cardiac failure) – overall (especially high in those with chromosomal abnormalities +/− heart disease)[a] | 1–5 % |
| Small bowel obstruction (early or late)[a] [Anastomotic stenosis/adhesion formation] | 1–5 % |
| Mortality – overall (depends on severity of other anomalies, rather than the duodenal obstruction itself) | 1–5 % |
| Mortality without surgery (may be up to 100 %) (lethal chromosomal abnormalities (e.g., trisomy 18) may preclude surgery)[a] | >80 % |
| *Rare significant/serious problems* | |
| Liver injury | 0.1–1 % |
| Subphrenic abscess | <0.1 % |
| Complete anastomotic (duodenotomy) breakdown | 0.1–1 % |
| *Less serious complications* | |
| Pain/tenderness | |
|   Acute (<4 weeks) | 5  20 % |
|   Chronic (>4 weeks) | <0.1 % |
| Intolerance of large meals (necessity for small frequent meals) | 20–50 % |
| Delayed gastric emptying (Universal for up to several weeks and probably universal to some extent for life) | >80 % |
| Wound scarring (poor cosmesis/wound deformity) | 1–5 % |
| Nasogastric tube[a] (sometimes for weeks) | 50–80 % |

[a]Dependent on underlying pathology, anatomy, surgical technique, and preferences
Important Note: Many of these complications are individually closely determined by the exact nature of the problem and surgery

## Major Complications

**Anastomotic leakage** is serious and occasionally not recognized early, leading to **intra-abdominal infection** and **abscess** formation. **Systemic infection and**

**multisystem failure** may then ensue. Concurrent cardiac anomalies may cause cardiac failure and increase mortality. **Bleeding** is rare and is usually controlled at surgery. **Wound infection** may occur and may lead to an incisional hernia. Wound **dehiscence** is rare. **Persistent duodenal obstruction** can result from inadequate division of a duodenal web or from anastomotic stenosis or functionally from severe dysmotility. **Severe gastroesophageal reflux** can be prolonged and may require fundoplication. **Small bowel obstruction** may occur from postoperative adhesions, even many years later. **Intravenous feeding** may be required if the stomach will not empty postoperatively.

---

**Consent and Risk Reduction**

**Main Points to Explain**

- GA risk
- Pain/discomfort
- Bleeding/hematoma*
- Infection (local/systemic)*
- Reflux problems
- Feeding problems
- Duodenal leakage
- Risk of other abdominal organ injury*
- Possible further surgery*
- Risks without surgery*
- Multisystem organ failure
- Death*

*Dependent on pathology, comorbidities, and surgery performed

---

# Surgery for Midgut Obstructions and Inflammation: Malrotation, Volvulus, Jejunoileal Obstruction, and Meconium Ileus

## Description

In any neonate with an intestinal obstruction, the objective of the operation is to define the problem and alleviate the obstruction. Resection of bowel may be required depending on the pathology and the degree of obstruction, ischemia, or necrosis present. For children, and especially neonates, a transverse muscle-cutting incision is typically used. There are few anatomical variations that affect the small bowel except for malrotation with Ladd's bands and a Meckel's diverticulum and other derivatives of the vitello intestinal duct. Malrotation is where the midgut loop fails to return to the abdominal cavity, with its normal rotation, between 10 and 12 weeks' gestation. A Meckel's diverticulum is a remnant of the vitellointestinal duct (the duct that runs from the yolk sac through the umbilicus to the apex of the midgut loop – where a Meckel's is situated), which can give rise to other problems as well as the well-known Meckel's diverticulum (see section "Surgery for Meckel's Diverticulum and Vitellointestinal Remnants"). In addition, small intestine atresias and meconium ileus are causes of small bowel obstruction in the newborn.

Malrotation is any departure from the usual final adult positioning of the gut within the abdomen. If a patient presents with an intestinal obstruction and hypovolemic shock as a newborn, the degree of malrotation is usually complete, with the second, third, and fourth parts of the duodenum running vertically down just to the right side of the midline, with the cecum and ascending colon running up just next to it, but to the left of the midline. These, together with all of the intervening small bowel, make up the midgut loop of the fetus. Where there is a complete malrotation, the midgut loop is closely applied to a central thick cordlike "universal mesentery" that hangs free in the abdomen. This contains the blood supply to all of the midgut loop, with the proximal small bowel vessels going to the right and the distal small bowel and large bowel vessels going to the left. As a result, this pendulum-like arrangement is very liable to twist on itself at the upper point of attachment, as the midgut fills with food for the first time. The baby presents with pain (screaming), hypovolemic shock, green bile vomiting (with or without blood), and the passage of blood rectally. Venous gangrene of the whole of the midgut loop – middle of the first part of the duodenum to just short of the splenic flexure of the colon – may occur. In the older child (or even adult), the degree of malrotation is often not as marked causing intermittent attacks of obstruction, with central abdominal pain and green bile vomiting. There is often a history of several such attacks, which appear to be able to resolve, presumably by the midgut untwisting, until the diagnosis is eventually made. Nevertheless, surgery is often as an emergency, because of a midgut volvulus. This can occur at any age, and patients have presented well into their 40s and older. The treatment is essentially the same as in babies (see Ladd's procedure below).

**Anatomical Points**

*Malrotation*

There are few anatomical variations that affect the small bowel except for Meckel's diverticulum and malrotation with Ladd's bands. A Meckel's diverticulum is a remnant of the vitellointestinal duct, which can give rise to other lesions as well as the well-known Meckel's diverticulum.

Malrotation can vary from complete failure to rotate to minor forms of maldescent of the cecum. In the fetus, the midgut loop is attached to the back wall of the abdomen at the middle of the second part of the duodenum and again just short of the splenic flexure. Between these two points, it is outside the abdomen in the umbilical cord. In the normal process of the midgut returning to the abdomen during the 10–12th week of gestation, the cecum and transverse colon rotate anterior to (over) the base of the small bowel mesentery with the cecum moving down to the RIF, as the duodenum rotates deep to it up into the LUQ. In that way, the root of the mesentery is attached diagonally across the whole of the abdomen on the longest

**Table 3.9** Surgery for midgut obstructions and inflammation estimated frequency of complications, risks, and consequences

| Complications, risks, and consequences | Estimated frequency |
| --- | --- |
| *Most significant/serious complications* | |
| Infection[a] | 5–20 % |
|   Subcutaneous | 5–20 % |
|   Intra-abdominal/pelvic (peritonitis; abscess) (especially in the ELBW; premature) | 5–20 % |
|   Systemic sepsis (especially in the ELBW; premature) | 2–5 % |
|   Hepatic portal sepsis (rare) | <0.1 % |
| Bleeding/hematoma formation[a] | |
|   Wound | 1–5 % |
|   Intra-abdominal | 0.1–1 % |
| Small bowel obstruction (postoperative early or late)[a] [Adhesion formation] | 1–5 % |
| Repeated further surgery[a] | 1–5 % |
| *Rare significant/serious problems* | |
| Perforation (spontaneous preoperative)[a] | 0.1–1 % |
| Anastomotic leakage[a] | 0.1–1 % |
| Fecal/enterocutaneous fistula[a] (very rare) | <0.1 % |
| Ureteric injury (very rare)[a] | <0.1 % |
| Multisystem organ failure (renal, pulmonary, cardiac failure) | 0.1–1 % |
| Mortality[a] | 0.1–1 % |
| Mortality <u>without</u> surgery (should surgery be refused)[a] | >80 % |
| *Less serious complications* | |
| Pain/tenderness | |
|   Acute (<4 weeks) | 5–20 % |
|   Chronic (>4 weeks) | <0.1 % |
| Paralytic ileus (peritonitis from preoperative perforation) | 20–30 % |
| Nerve parasthesia | 0.1–1 % |
| Wound scarring (poor cosmesis/wound deformity)[a] | 1–5 % |
| Nasogastric tube[a] | 1–5 % |
| Wound drain tube(s)[a] | 1–5 % |

[a]Dependent on underlying pathology, anatomy, surgical technique, and preferences

Note: ELBW extremely low-birth-weight newborn, <1,000 g

Important Note: Many of these complications are individually closely determined by the exact nature of the problem and surgery. The extent and underlying disease will alter the relative risks

attachment possible. If, as the intestine returns to the abdomen, it fails to rotate, then it simply hangs in the abdomen attached as it was in the fetus. Ladd's bands represent the course the colon should have taken and therefore stretch across the duodenum.

**Mirror image malrotation**, although thought to be rare, is now more frequently detected antenatally in association with left atrial isomerism, with situs inversus abdominus. The gut is the mirror image of normal, but is also frequently malrotated. A barium meal after birth confirms the situs inversus with the malrotation, and the patient then undergoes a mirror image Ladd's procedure – often laparoscopically.

*Malrotation: Complications of the Disease*

**Volvulus,** usually of the entire midgut, occurs clockwise when viewed from in front. The vascular supply will be compromised to a varying degree and may cause venous then arterial infarction. In addition, the malrotation may be associated with duodenal obstruction from congenital bands running from the ascending colon across the front of the duodenum (Ladd's bands). Volvulus occurs in the baby, while partial obstructions or volvulus can occur in the older child. If left too long, the patient will die of hypovolemic shock and/or venous gangrene of the whole of the midgut loop – middle of the second part of the duodenum to just short of the splenic flexure of the colon. The most significant complication is ischemic infarction of the midgut loop with subsequent death or years of parenteral nutrition followed by a gut transplant. With an established volvulus, death is inevitable without surgery.

In the premature it is very difficult to differentiate between necrotizing enterocolitis (see 46.10) and a midgut volvulus. Both have the same presentation, viz., hypovolemic shock and bowel obstruction. But, NEC is treated expectantly, initially, which would be disastrous where there is volvulus of the midgut loop. An ultrasound of the upper abdominal vasculature and the first few loops of bowel may well differentiate, whereas a plain X-ray may not. But, if there is any doubt, an emergency laparotomy should be performed without delay.

*Malrotation: The Surgery and Its Complications*

**Ladd's Procedure:** The surgery for malrotation with or without volvulus is done as soon as possible to try to minimize gut loss. As for all obstructions to the small bowel in the neonate, an upper transverse muscle-cutting approach is used. Any volvulus is untwisted anticlockwise as you look at it. Ladd's bands (fibrous bands running from the ascending colon across the duodenum) are divided, allowing the colon to be moved further to the left, exposing the root of the mesentery and the duodenum. The thick rope-like "universal mesentery" is splayed/teased open, so that the vessels to the duodenum and jejunum can be moved to the right, and the vessels to the terminal ileum, ascending colon, and transverse colon can be moved to the left. In this way the corresponding intestine can be moved with the vessels as far away from the midline as possible. Normal anatomy cannot be established as the ileocecal vessels that normally run down to the RIF now run a very short distance to the ascending colon, which is in the high midline. The most mobile parts of the rest of the small intestine are then placed back over the raw area created by splitting the mesentery, so that they will form adhesions to that area, hopefully preventing further twisting. The cecum is placed in the LIF and an appendectomy is usually carried out.

**Laparoscopic Ladd's Procedure**: The procedure can now be performed laparoscopically, even in the presence of volvulus, and is being performed more and more commonly with time. Obtaining an adequate window to obtain an adequate view is often difficult when the gut is distended, so conversion to an open procedure is not uncommon when volvulus has occurred.

**Complications of the Disease:** If there is gangrenous bowel, then it has to be resected, hopefully, without losing the entire midgut loop, as this will be essentially lethal, without prolonged TPN, +/− SB transplantation. If surgery is delayed, then the patient may be irretrievable.

**Complications of the Surgery:** Short-term problems are survival of the child and the intestine and then leaking anastomoses. The dissection in the mesentery often injures lacteals, which will produce a temporary chylous ascites. A short-to medium-chain fat dietary substitute or parenteral nutrition for 4–6 weeks may be useful if prolonged ileus occurs.

Longer term, the deliberate placing of the mobile part of the small bowel into the raw dissected mesentery will lead to extensive adhesions. While this will diminish the tendency to a recurrence of any volvulus, it does increase the incidence of adhesive obstruction, so that there is a 20–30 % lifetime risk of an adhesive bowel obstruction (Murphy et al. 2006).

### *Jejunoileal Obstruction in the Newborn*

**Jejunoileal obstruction in the newborn** is predominantly associated with an atresia probably caused by a complete interruption to the blood flow to the intestine in the fetus. This leads to loss of the intestine. Because the fetal bowel contains no organisms, the dead bowel disappears, and the two blind ends seal themselves. Intestinal atresias take various forms, from loss of the lumen only to a significant gap, or multiple atresias with small remaining segments – "a string of sausages" (Federici et al. 2003). Incomplete obstruction associated with stenosis is rare (but does occur in the duodenum). Jejunoileal obstructions are rarely associated with other congenital anomalies. Unless the atresia is associated with a significant or lethal loss of bowel, the long-term outlook is usually good. In those with a very proximal jejunal atresia, the degree of dilatation of the proximal bowel may be grotesque so that disparity between it and the distal bowel is a major issue.

### *Complications of the Disease*

### *Jejunal Atresia*

Proximal to a jejunal atresia, the obstructed intestine undergoes massive dilation and becomes inert (thought to be due to ischemic changes in the antimesenteric wall plus the back-pressure effect). These dramatic changes are easily detected on antenatal ultrasound. At birth, an X-ray will show relatively few grossly distended loops of bowel. As with all small bowel obstructions in the newborn, if left untreated, the proximal intestine will progressively distend and will eventually perforate or infarct with subsequent peritonitis and death.

**The Surgery:** In all small bowel atresias, the proximal intestine becomes distended, and the distal intestine becomes shrunken and unused. The more proximal the atresia, the more marked the upstream distension, giving rise to a gross disparity in size especially in proximal jejunal atresias, so that anastomoses are difficult. Where possible the most distended part of the intestine (the distal end of the proximal part) is resected, thereby presenting a less distended part to be anastomosed. Jejunal atresias are frequently close to the DJ flexure, limiting the surgeon's ability to resect all of the distended bowel. Nevertheless, the most grossly dilated bowel is resected, where possible. The rest of the distended proximal intestine is tailored to a narrower tube (by discarding the floppy antimesenteric part) and is anastomosed with its end anastomosed to a longitudinal incision made into the antimesenteric border of the distal (contracted and unused) small bowel – the so-called end-to-back anastomosis used in all anastomosis of the small and large intestine where there has been a congenital small or large bowel obstruction. The end-to-back anastomosis allows a larger than normal proximal intestine to be anastomosed to a smaller than normal distal intestine. As for all intestinal anastomoses in the newborn, a single-layer interrupted absorbable suturing technique is usually used. In North America, however, stapling is often used especially for the tailoring procedure in jejunal atresia. Where there are multiple atresias, resection and multiple anastomoses may be required. Occasionally, a temporary proximal stoma may be used to protect multiple distal anastomoses while they seal and heal.

**Complications of the Surgery**: There are two common postoperative issues. The first is that the long tailoring suture line may leak, and/or stricture, and secondly the proximal intestine will take a long time to recover its motility after the prenatal ischemic damage (that caused the atresia in the first place) and the long-tailored anastomosis. Therefore, these babies often require IV nutrition for weeks.

*Ileal Atresia*

This is less common, but has its own unique problems. In one specific circumstance where there is a distal ileal atresia, the blood supply to the distal ileum is derived from an ascending branch of the ileocolic artery running back up the small bowel from the ileocecal junction. So, if there is a gap in the mesentery anywhere in the distal ileum supplied by this vessel, then the intestine is free to twist around the artery, and if it does, it creates the appearance of an "apple-peel atresia." As with jejunal atresia, the proximal intestine will dilate, but not as markedly as for jejunal atresias.

**The Surgery**: Uncomplicated atresias can occur anywhere in between these two sites (the grossly distended proximal jejunal atresia and the distal ileum's apple peel). Then, the surgery is far more straightforward; the most distended part of the proximal intestine is resected and an end-to-end anastomosis carried out. Recovery times are far shorter, but still take a few days. The apple-peel atresia's tenuous blood supply makes it difficult to straighten out the intestine and reanastomose the ends, as the part that has been spiraled around the artery may lose its blood supply as it is straightened. Therefore, partial resection of this intestine is frequently necessary to ensure a good blood supply to both ends.

Long-term complications for jejunal and ileal atresias are few. Adhesive obstruction occurs in approximately 5 % and usually within 2 years of the surgery. Where there has been an abdominal wall defect, the adhesive obstruction rate is higher (van Eijck et al. 2008). Rarely the loss of intestine is critical. If it is, then long-term parenteral nutrition is required, while enteral feeding is gradually established. Hopefully, the residual gut gradually adapts to enable full enteral feeding. In the newborn, the gut is still growing and appears to be able to compensate for some of the loss of length, as well as being able to undergo mucosal adaptation.

If, however, the residual gut is not long enough to support life, then there are gut lengthening procedures (where the gut is split longitudinally and then reanastomosed end-to-end) or interposition procedures (that slow the transit time) that have been used. They have met with mixed success. The "multiple step" procedure is now gaining popularity (proceedings of the World Congress of Surgery, Adelaide, 2008). This is a procedure where there are multiple incisions made into the side of the gut for just over half of its circumference, and then those incisions are closed longitudinally. The gut is then lengthened rather like a paper chain. This procedure appears to increase transit time, and as the residual narrowed gut dilates, it increases the absorptive surface area as well. Initial results would suggest that this is more successful than the older procedures.

If the terminal ileum has to be resected, then vitamin $B_{12}$ absorption will be poor. If the resection is carried out in the neonate, however, then passive absorption appears to compensate (Ooi et al. 1992) to a far greater extent than in the adult, so that serum levels of $B_{12}$ are usually normal. The Schilling test will be abnormal. If the serum levels are normal, supplements are not necessary in childhood, but levels should be checked. When such an affected female becomes pregnant, however, the fetus requires folate and $B_{12}$ at levels that cannot then be supplied by a normal diet for this mother, so that females who have lost the terminal ileum need to be aware of the extra requirement during pregnancy.

## Meconium ileus

**Meconium ileus** is a neonatal intestinal obstruction that occurs in 14 % of newborns with cystic fibrosis (Efrati et al. 2010) (but obstruction may occur in older cystic fibrosis patients when it is known as "meconium ileus equivalent"). It is due to viscid intestinal mucus causing obstruction of the small bowel in the distal ileum, with proximal intestinal dilatation. On antenatal ultrasound, this dilatation can be detected, and it is often accompanied by echogenic bowel at that time.

Some 10 % of cystic fibrosis patients will present at birth with this form of bowel obstruction, approximately 1:20,000 live births (Rescorla et al. 1998). The obstruction in meconium ileus may be a simple intraluminal small bowel obstruction (SBO) from inspissation of mucus, which becomes a concrete-like series of plugs in the ileum. Or, the back-pressure from this obstruction may cause proximal segmental volvulus with loss of intestine in the fetus. Or, the obstruction may cause a proximal perforation and leak of meconium before birth. In the latter, the baby is born with meconium peritonitis, where the abdominal viscera are fixed in highly inflamed adhesions from the sterile peritonitis (Rescorla et al. 1998).

*Conservative Treatment*

With meconium ileus, as above, ischemia, perforation, sepsis, and respiratory difficulties from abdominal distension may supervene at birth. If there is an uncomplicated meconium obstruction, repeated contrast enemas with gastrografin (which contains a detergent) may clear the obstruction, but laparotomy is often required because the obstruction may not clear fast enough to alleviate abdominal distension and respiratory distress.

*Surgical Correction*

At laparotomy for the intestinal obstruction, resection of the most distended part of the intestine is performed if there is a simple distal luminal obstruction. The residual distal ileum is then flushed through with normal saline until the colon is seen to clear. If this is ineffective, then a temporary stoma of the type that allows the distal intestine to be flushed is used. If there has been a proximal volvulus, then the ischemic gut is resected if it is still present. If it has already disappeared, the resultant atresia is dealt with as above. If cystic fibrosis has been complicated by meconium peritonitis before birth, the adhesions are usually dense and inflamed. Then a temporary stoma is often used. A follow-up laparotomy is carried out 4–6 weeks later when the inflammation has subsided. The areas of adhesive obstruction can be corrected and the stoma closed. Another cause of segmental volvulus can occur around a persistent vitellointestinal band connecting the umbilicus with the small bowel at the site of a Meckel's diverticulum (see section 46.12).

**Perspective**

See Table 3.9. The complications of operations for small bowel obstruction depend on the initial pathology for which the procedure was performed. Death from hypovolemic shock and/or midgut necrosis and gangrene is well recorded if the surgery for midgut volvulus is delayed. In the very premature that have a volvulus, the diagnosis can be missed as these babies are thought to have necrotizing enterocolitis (NEC), which is much more common and presents with a similar initial picture. The two diseases may be combined, as the midgut loop develops gangrene.

A serious complication of any gut resection is an anastomotic leakage, the risk of which is increased by more distal obstruction of any cause or perforation with peritonitis. So, it is vital to alleviate any significant obstruction distal to any anastomosis. Therefore, in any baby with an atresia, it is mandatory to follow the distal bowel to the pelvic floor, preferably flushing it with warm saline at the same time to ensure its patency, as there may well be multiple atresias. The consequence of an anastomotic leakage is contamination of the peritoneal cavity leading to generalized peritonitis or intra-abdominal abscess formation, anywhere and everywhere in the neonate. Surprisingly, however, the neonate tolerates this well, and if a drain is placed through the wound after a leak is suspected, then the leak will often spontaneously close as peristalsis distal to the anastomosis becomes established. The risks of an anastomotic leakage are reduced by ensuring good blood supply to the bowel ends, minimal tension, and no factors contraindicating an anastomosis.

The risks of wound infection, small bowel obstruction, enterocutaneous fistula and short bowel syndrome are significant, but fortunately uncommon complications, and are seen more often after necrotizing enterocolitis (see section 46.10). After a Ladd's procedure, the lifetime risk of an adhesive SBO may be as high as 20–30 % (Murphy et al. 2006). After a tailored jejunal atresia correction, SBO may be as high as 20 %, with reoperation in the first few weeks of life. The risk of short-gut syndrome depends on the type of lesion and the amount of small bowel resected or lost before birth, as does the risk of nutritional deficiency.

Ileus is common, but usually short lived (except in jejunal and duodenal atresias), being dependent on the amount of gut manipulation and inflammation. Incisional herniae are usually minor and often close themselves when surgery is performed on the newborn. Older age groups carry a higher risk of non-closure.

## Major Complications

The type of complication is dependent on the surgery required and the extent of the disease entity present. Detorsion of a volvulus may be associated with **reperfusion-type injury** with release of ischemic products with **shock, hypotension,** and **sepsis. Perforation of the bowel** is associated with **intraperitoneal sepsis,** including **abscess formation** and **wound infection.** Where used, **anastomotic leakage** may occur. **Enterocutaneous or internal fistula** may arise. Adhesion formation and **small bowel obstruction** may occur which can be recurrent. **Systemic sepsis** may occur and may lead to **multisystem organ failure** and **death.**

**Consent and Risk Reduction**

**Main Points to Explain**

- GA risk
- Pain/discomfort
- Bleeding/hematoma*
- Infection (local/systemic)*
- Feeding problems
- Risk of other abdominal organ injury*
- Possible further surgery*
- Risks without surgery*
- Multisystem organ failure
- Death*

- **\*Dependent on pathology, comorbidities, and surgery performed**

# Surgery for Necrotizing Enterocolitis

**Necrotizing enterocolitis (NEC)** is a life-threatening condition of uncertain etiology, which mainly affects the very premature baby (Albanese et al. 1998). It is associated with ischemic damage to any part of the bowel, from the DJ flexure to the rectum. The most common sites of disease are the terminal ileum and the sigmoid colon. It acts as a gas gangrene of the bowel wall with partial- or full-thickness necrosis of the intestine for short segments, or all of the bowel, or anything in between. Gas collects in between the layers of the intestinal wall and shows up on X-ray as pneumatosis before perforation. When there has been full-thickness necrosis, perforation will be demonstrated by a pneumoperitoneum and further sepsis.

The initial treatment of NEC is broad-spectrum antibiotics, IV feeding, and gut rest. Once the bowel is necrotic, subsequent bacterial leakage, infection, and perforation will occur, possibly causing death. The disease can be remarkably rapid in its progress. The indications for surgery are obvious perforation, increasing difficulty in ventilation because the abdomen is so tense, increasing systemic sepsis, thrombocytopenia, and inability to control the unstable patient. But, before any of these occur, attempts are made to treat the patient with broad-spectrum antibiotics, IV feeding, and gut rest.

## Anatomical Points

The extent of gut affected largely determines the amount and type of resection, but based on the relatively constant anatomical blood supply. However, in situations where malrotation or other congenital anomalies, such as situs inversus, exist, the blood supply and anatomy can be considerably distorted.

## Complications of the Disease

NEC affects approximately 5 % of the premature, which in turn accounts for 1 % of newborns. Of those >1,000 g birth weight, conservative management with IV antibiotics and IV feeding leads to a 70 % recovery without surgery. For those <1,000 g, the extremely low birth weight (ELBW), the disease is remarkably rapid and affects large segments, if not all of the small bowel.

In the ELBW neonates, the occurrence of generalized peritonitis occurs early so that the patient is often not fit for major surgery. In that scenario, placement of peritoneal drains will buy time in which to try to stabilize the baby before a laparotomy. Occasionally, no further surgery is necessary as the perforation(s) close themselves. Nevertheless, late surgery for fistula, stricture, and obstruction is the rule.

Many of the complications listed under complications of the surgery are really complications of the disease, e.g., strictures, malabsorption, and recurrent obstruction.

**Table 3.10** Surgery for necrotizing enterocolitis estimated frequency of complications, risks, and consequences

| Complications, risks, and consequences | Estimated frequency |
|---|---|
| *Most significant/serious complications* | |
| Infection[a] | 5–20 % |
|   Subcutaneous | 5–20 % |
|   Intra-abdominal/pelvic (peritonitis; abscess) (especially in the ELBW; premature) | 5–20 % |
|   Systemic sepsis (especially in the ELBW; premature) | 2–5 % |
|   Hepatic portal sepsis (rare) | <0.1 % |
| Bleeding/hematoma formation[a] | |
|   Wound | 1–5 % |
|   Intra-abdominal | 0.1–1 % |
| Small bowel obstruction (postoperative early or late; stricture formation)[a] [Adhesion formation] | 1–5 % |
| Repeated further surgery[a] | 1–5 % |
| Intellectual impairment[a] (especially ELBW) | 50–80 % |
| *Rare significant/serious problems* | |
| Perforation (spontaneous preoperative)[a] | 0.1–1 % |
| Anastomotic leakage[a] | 0.1–1 % |
| Temporary stoma(s)[a] | 0.1–1 % |
| Fecal/enterocutaneous fistula(e)[a] (very rare) | <0.1 % |
| Ureteric injury (very rare)[a] | <0.1 % |
| Liver failure from prolonged cholestasis[a] | 0.1–1 % |
| Nutritional deficiency $B_{12}$ malabsorption[a] | 0.1–1 % |
| Wound breakdown[a] | 0.1–1 % |
| Multisystem organ failure (renal, pulmonary, cardiac failure) | 0.1–1 % |
| Mortality[a] (especially ELBW) | 50–80 % |
| Mortality[a] (term infants) | 5–20 % |
| Mortality without surgery (should surgery be refused)[a] | >80 % |
| *Less serious complications* | |
| Pain/tenderness | |
|   Acute (<4 weeks) | 5–20 % |
|   Chronic (>4 weeks) | <0.1 % |
| Paralytic ileus (peritonitis from preoperative perforation) | 20–30 % |
| Nerve parasthesia | 0.1–1 % |
| Wound scarring (poor cosmesis/wound deformity)[a] | 1–5 % |
| Nasogastric tube[a] | 1–5 % |
| Wound drain tube(s)[a] | 1–5 % |

[a]Dependent on underlying pathology, anatomy, surgical technique, and preferences
Note: ELBW extremely low-birth-weight newborn, <1,000 g
Important Note: Many of these complications are individually closely determined by the exact nature of the problem and surgery. The extent and underlying disease will alter the relative risks

## The Surgery

### Open Laparotomy for Perforation, Sepsis, and Ischemic Gangrene

Laparotomy and gut resection are reserved for where there is failure of conservative treatment or for obvious perforation with sepsis, for prolonged and frank bowel obstruction, or for where the patient is deteriorating but could still tolerate a laparotomy. In these circumstances, there is nearly always more disease than expected, often with obvious segments of gangrenous intestine with or without multiple perforations.

### For Those Unfit for Laparotomy

In the ELBW neonate, the disease often progresses so rapidly that there is systemic collapse. In that situation there is still controversy as to whether or not an immediate laparotomy should be carried out or drains should be inserted in the ICU with analgesia. At the moment, the consensus is that drains should be used to gain time followed by a laparotomy when the neonate is fitter. Others would stop at the drainage alone and wait and see if the intestine will seal, and gut continuity will be restored. The literature claims that this may occur in up to 30 % of patients treated in this manner, but local experience has met with virtually no success.

### Spontaneous Perforation of the Small Bowel

There is a group of growth restricted (too small for gestational age at birth) neonates that develop a so-called spontaneous perforation of the terminal ileum (Messina et al. 2009). This appears to be the only affected area of the gut. Often there is a distal microcolon where the colon is small, shut down, and dysmotile. This appears to cause a localized back-pressure perforation in the last part of the small bowel and small areas of muscle loss in the intestine elsewhere. Clinically, the abdomen is soft, but distended, abdominal X-ray demonstrates a huge pneumoperitoneum, and initially the neonate is stable with no systemic effects. This perforation occurs in the first few days of life, whereas NEC usually only occurs several days if not weeks after birth. This local perforation is treated very differently to those with gross and frank widespread NEC. This localized lesion can be treated through a minilaparotomy in the RIF, creating a small local stoma to allow the small bowel to work and to allow the neonate to be fed enterally while waiting for the colon to start to work.

## Complications of the Surgery

Neonates >1,000 g tolerate laparotomies and major gut resections well, even in the presence of gross intra-abdominal sepsis. For neonates >1,000 g who undergo surgery (30 % of those that develop the disease), there is a 5–10 % perioperative mortality, with the potential for intellectual morbidity in those that survive.

But, in those <1,000 g (the extremely low-birth-weight group [ELBW], usually 24–26 weeks' gestation), there is no hard figure for how many will get NEC and how many will survive without surgery (on conservative Rx, e.g., drainage only – see above), but for those that go to surgery, approximately 60 % will die soon after the surgery because there is so much dead bowel that nothing can be done, and the abdomen is just closed again. For those that survive surgery, 70 % will have moderate to severe intellectual handicap(s) (Chacko et al. 1999). The brain damage is thought to arise from gross pre- and postoperative vascular instability with large shifts in blood pressure, especially in the central and intracranial venous systems, accompanied by large shifts in blood gases. After counseling before surgery, parents nearly always insist on the laparotomy despite this poor prognosis, which may leave them with a severely handicapped child.

### Intra- and Postoperative Hemorrhage

In the ELBW group, there is little supporting stroma for blood vessels to the intestine and especially blood vessels in the liver. The liver is also very soft and is disproportionately large, often well down in the RIF, overlying the terminal ileum, one of the most frequently diseased areas in NEC. Therefore, the liver can be easily lacerated, even by simple retraction, and will not stop bleeding. Therefore, in the ELBW patient who requires a laparotomy, avoid entering the abdomen high on the right.

### Liver Failure from Prolonged Cholestasis

**Liver failure from prolonged cholestasis** is a major problem after major gut resection in premature neonates. Contributing factors are prematurity, multiple abdominal procedures, a gut that will not tolerate enteral feeding because of prolonged ileus, prolonged parenteral nutrition, and intra-abdominal sepsis with or without systemic sepsis.

### Nutritional Deficiency $B_{12}$ Malabsorption

Although the terminal ileum is frequently removed, the incidence of a low serum $B_{12}$ is actually low. The Schilling test is abnormal. So, it appears that if the terminal ileum is removed as a premature baby, then passive absorption takes over to a degree that maintains serum levels (Ooi et al. 1992). But, be careful to warn the mother and the female child who has lost the terminal ileum (when older) that although the patient's $B_{12}$ and folate may be normal, absorption is such that it will decompensate during a pregnancy. Therefore, the fetus of a mother who has lost her terminal ileum as a baby is at risk of intrauterine brain damage, unless aggressive supplementation is carried out in that mother.

### Wound Breakdown

**Wound breakdown** can occur especially in the very premature. Because of the poor resistance to infection in this age group and the major difficulties in maintaining adequate nutrition (where there is intra-abdominal sepsis), wound infection is very common. Superficial breakdown of the wound is also very common. Surprisingly wound dehiscence is rare, and the wounds gradually close.

### Stricture (Early and Late) and Obstruction

Strictures occur because of the disease itself. They are not apparent at the emergency laparotomy as the process is one of gangrene at that time. These diseased areas that are left behind then scar and stricture down. Presentation is bimodal: there is an acute presentation due to inflammation, necrosis, and swelling causing an obstruction, which may settle down with conservative treatment, but often goes on to a true stricture within days or weeks of the laparotomy, and/or there is a later presentation (up to years afterward but usually within a year) where a mature fibrous stricture forms. This will not relent.

### Fistula(e)

Fistulae are seen often after surgery. They are more common after primary anastomoses. Surprisingly most settle on conservative management: nil by mouth and IV feeding. This does not need a laparotomy straightaway and does not mandate that drains should be placed at the time of the initial surgery, as this appears to increase the fistula rate.

### Perspective

See Table 3.10. Death and brain damage are likely outcomes in the extremely low-birth-weight (ELBW) group. Anastomotic leak and anastomotic stricture are common (diseased ends to the bowel anastomosed, when every effort is being made to preserve bowel length). These problems are difficult to avoid, as the whole of the gut has poor perfusion, which is the presumed trigger for the disease. Temporary stomas are therefore frequently used to avoid an anastomosis in a patient who is in multi-organ failure, who has a tense abdomen and has to be ventilated at high pressures. Possibly simple drainage should be used, but that decision is made on a case-by-case basis. Short bowel syndrome may be a long-term issue. The extent of preoperative obstruction, ischemia, or perforation and contamination is a significant factor in the severity of postoperative complications and consequences. NEC is associated with relatively more severe complications overall, including nonsurgically related delayed neural development, as the disease occurs predominantly in the premature, which itself leads to a higher risk of intellectual impairment. The presence of other anomalies, and chronic lung disease, associated with prematurity may greatly influence the incidence of multisystem organ failure and mortality.

### Major Complications

**Anastomotic leakage, spontaneous perforation, abscess formation,** and **abdominal sepsis** may lead to **systemic sepsis, multisystem organ failure,** and **death. Repeated further surgery,** with or without **small bowel obstruction,** may occur. **Mental and intellectual disabilities,** especially in the very low-birth-weight groups, are serious longer-term problems that may develop. **Bleeding** intra- and postoperatively can occur. **Liver failure** may supervene. **Nutritional disturbances,** including malnutrition, may result if large lengths of bowel are resected.

**Consent and Risk Reduction**

**Main Points to Explain**

- GA risk
- Pain/discomfort
- Bleeding/hematoma*
- Infection (local/systemic)*
- Feeding problems
- Nutritional deficiency
- Risk of other abdominal organ injury*
- Later liver problems
- Possible further surgery*
- Risks without surgery*
- Multisystem organ failure
- Death*

**\*Dependent on pathology, comorbidities, and surgery performed**

## Surgery for Hirschsprung's Disease

### Description

The failure of complete migration of neural crest cells to form the submucous and myenteric plexuses at the distal end of the bowel leads to the aganglionosis of Hirschsprung's disease. As there is failure of these cells to reach the end of the hindgut, Hirschsprung's disease is the absence of ganglion cells from just above the dentate line back up the intestine for a variable distance, to the point where the neural crest cell migration ceased. In 70 % of patients, the aganglionosis will involve part of the rectum, the whole of the rectum, or the rectum and sigmoid; the remaining 30 % will have longer segments. The disease occurs in approximately 1 in 5,000 live births.

The final diagnosis is a tissue diagnosis, not an imaging diagnosis, so biopsies have to be taken. Bowel obstruction may be significant, and perforation can occur, especially if enterocolitis supervenes. The aim of surgery is to resect the aganglionic segment of colon and anastomose ganglionic bowel to the anus, just above the dentate line. Occasionally, the resected segment may involve the entire colon and very rarely may involve large parts of the small bowel to the extent that survival is not possible. The disease is more common in trisomy 21 (Ieiri et al. 2009) and other rarer chromosomal abnormalities, e.g., a 13q deletion (Khong et al. 1994); there are familial cases and known gene defects strongly suggesting that there is a hereditary predisposition to the disease.

### Surgery

The surgery for Hirschsprung's disease has traditionally been a staged procedure with a temporary colostomy, later the definitive procedure, and then closure of the colostomy. But, total correction at birth as a one-stage procedure is becoming more popular. Many would do the definitive procedure as a combined laparotomy and transanal approach, but a purely transanal neonatal approach without a colostomy or laparotomy is now also gaining favor. When a laparotomy is combined with a perineal procedure, there are three ways of doing the operation: the "Soave," the "Duhamel," or the "Swenson." All have their proponents, the basic aim remains: to remove the aganglionic section and partly destroy the internal sphincter action and bring ganglionic bowel down to just above the dentate line.

*Emergency Colostomy*

Where the neonate is too ill to undergo a definitive procedure (e.g., where there is a life-threatening Hirschsprung's colitis), an initial colostomy is used but must be in ganglionic bowel (monitored by frozen section).

*Routine Colostomy*

With a staged approach to the disease, plain X-ray and contrast studies may help to determine where the transition from aganglionic to ganglionic bowel occurs. Often, these are not accurate. If a colostomy is to be used as a preliminary to an interval definitive procedure, then frozen section biopsies are taken to ensure that the colon is placed in ganglionic bowel. Seromuscular biopsies are taken from the peritoneal reflection (to prove the diagnosis) and then another at the apparent transition zone, where there is a change in caliber from dilated proximal to narrowed distal intestine. If the transition zone is confirmed, then a separated double-ended stoma, 5–10 cm proximal to that transition zone, is formed, as that transition zone will not be fully ganglionic. This will usually be in the LIF (as 70 % of patients will have disease up to the rectosigmoid) so the surgery is initiated through a muscle-splitting incision. If there are no ganglion cells, then more and more proximal biopsies are needed. Extending the transverse incision across the abdomen will suffice, as the whole of the abdomen can be reached from a low transverse incision in the neonate. It is advisable to avoid a colostomy in the transverse colon as they frequently prolapse, sometimes within months.

*Definitive Staged Procedure*

Again the choice is operator dependent, using one of the three forms of pull-through procedure. The "Swenson" is a low anterior resection, eviscerating the rectal stump to complete the anastomosis outside the anus. The posterior end of the excision goes down to and includes the posterior part of the internal sphincter. The "Duhamel" is a procedure that brings normally innervated intestine down behind a rectal stump converting them both into one large chamber, again to a level that destroys the back of the internal sphincter. The "Soave" is an endorectal pull-through procedure removing the mucosa but leaving the external muscle layers of the anorectum intact as a sleeve (but cut down the back to avoid stricture), again down to the dentate line. All three of these have been used as a one-stage procedure in the neonate.

*Neonatal One-Stage Transanal Approach*

The dissection starts through the anus, elevating the mucosa off the underlying smooth muscle from just above the dentate line and then converting to full thickness at 5–6 cm (the level of the pelvic floor and above the ureters). Full-thickness frozen sections are taken as the bowel is eviscerated through the anus, until such time as ganglionic bowel is reached. If the length of the intestine to be eviscerated through the anal canal does not get into the ganglionic bowel (the limit of simple eviscera-tion through the anus is approximately 30 cm), then laparoscopy with 3 mm instru-ments can be employed to divide the mesocolon to a point where ganglionic bowel can then be eviscerated through the anus.

Full-thickness frozen sections are taken at points at the predicted transition zone, or at any change in caliber, and continue to be taken until the pathologist is sure that there are ganglion cells. The ganglionic bowel is then anastomosed to the dentate line outside the anus. This is done as a one-stage procedure, and the baby is often feeding fully the next day! If the surgeon plans to do a transanal "Soave" (second stage) after doing an emergency colostomy in a sick neonate with Hirschsprung's enterocolitis (first stage), then a colostomy in the LIF is too low, as it will interfere with the mobilization of the colon from below. Then, for the emergency colostomy, its placement should be far more proximal (e.g., at the splenic flexure), so that the Soave can be done later.

A neonatal "Duhamel" can be done as a combined perineal laparoscopic proce-dure using a stapler from below.

**Anatomical Points**

The extent of the aganglionic segment(s) is variable in different individuals, and this needs to be determined using biopsy during surgery. Other anomalies or genetic defects may alter the anatomy.

**Complications of the Disease**

*Early*

The worst complication is Hirschsprung's enterocolitis. This can be the presenting condition for these babies, and in cases where the diagnosis has been missed, this can be the presentation in the older child. If this occurs as the primary presentation, then the disease must be treated with broad-spectrum antibiotics and a colostomy with frozen section control. Once under control, the definitive surgery can then take the normal pathway(s). Enterocolitis (Teitelbaum et al. 1998) is not limited to those who have yet to undergo surgery, as a few will continue to have bouts of enteroco-litis for years after the surgery. Hold up in the intestine is blamed for these recurring attacks, whether this is due to inherent sluggishness in the residual disease or the result of inadequate surgery is unclear.

**Table 3.11** Surgery for Hirschsprung's disease estimated frequency of complications, risks, and consequences

| Complications, risks, and consequences | Estimated frequency |
|---|---|
| ***Most significant/serious complications*** | |
| Infection[a] | 5–20 % |
| Subcutaneous | 5–20 % |
| Intra-abdominal/pelvic (peritonitis; abscess) | 5–20 % |
| Systemic sepsis (especially in the ELBW; premature) | 2–5 % |
| Hepatic portal sepsis (rare) | <0.1 % |
| Bleeding/hematoma formation[a] | |
| Wound | 1–5 % |
| Intra-abdominal | 0.1–1 % |
| Small bowel obstruction (postoperative early or late; stricture formation)[a] [Adhesion formation] | 1–5 % |
| Repeated further surgery[a] | 1–5 % |
| Stomal problems[a] (prolapse; intussusception) | 5–20 % |
| Stricture formation[a] (anorectal) | 5–20 % |
| Fecal retention (peculiar to the Duhamel)[a] | 50–80 % |
| Fecal incontinence and fecalomas retention[a] | 50–80 % |
| Hirschsprung's enterocolitis[a] | 5–20 % |
| Peri-anal excoriation[a] | 50–80 % |
| Intellectual impairment[a] (especially ELBW) | 50–80 % |
| ***Rare significant/serious problems*** | |
| Perforation (spontaneous preoperative)[a] | 0.1–1 % |
| Anastomotic leakage[a] | 0.1–1 % |
| Temporary stoma(s)[a] | 0.1–1 % |
| Bowel injury (operative serious)[a] | 0.1–1 % |
| Ureteric injury (very rare)[a] | <0.1 % |
| Fecal/enterocutaneous fistula(e)[a] (very rare) | <0.1 % |
| Liver failure from prolonged cholestasis[a] | 0.1–1 % |
| Nutritional deficiency $B_{12}$ malabsorption[a] | 0.1–1 % |
| Wound breakdown[a] | 0.1–1 % |
| Multisystem organ failure (renal, pulmonary, cardiac failure) | 0.1–1 % |
| Mortality[a] (especially ELBW) | 50–80 % |
| Mortality[a] (term infants) | 5–20 % |
| Mortality without surgery (should surgery be refused)[a] | >80 % |
| ***Less serious complications*** | |
| Pain/tenderness | |
| Acute (<4 weeks) | 5–20 % |
| Chronic (>4 weeks) | <0.1 % |
| Paralytic ileus (peritonitis from preoperative perforation) | 20–30 % |
| Nerve parasthesia | 0.1–1 % |
| Wound scarring (poor cosmesis/wound deformity)[a] | 1–5 % |
| Nasogastric tube[a] | 1–5 % |
| Wound drain tube(s)[a] | 1–5 % |

[a]Dependent on underlying pathology, anatomy, surgical technique, and preferences

Note: ELBW extremely low-birth-weight newborn, <1,000 g

Important Note: Many of these complications are individually closely determined by the exact nature of the problem and surgery. The extent and underlying disease will alter the relative risks

**Complications of the Surgery**

See Table 3.11. If a staged procedure is used, then there are complications of the stoma, of the later definitive procedure, and the closure of a stoma. If a primary neonatal procedure is used, then the stomal complications do not occur, but stricture rates for the neonatal transanal approach are higher (but respond well to dilatation). Ischemia of the stoma occurs in 1–5 % leading to 'die-back' of the stoma and refashioning. Intussusception of the stoma is uncommon if placed in the sigmoid or low descending colon, but frequently occurs if the stoma is placed in the transverse colon. Postoperative obstruction and stricture formation rates depend on the procedure employed. A stricture rate of up to 5–20 % (more likely in the Swenson, and especially the transanal Soave) can occur, but these strictures can be reversed by almost routine anal canal dilatations, giving a good long-term result.

Later problems include incontinence and fecalomas, with overflow incontinence. Fecal retention occurs in all forms of surgery for Hirschsprung's disease if an aggressive stance is not taken to make sure that the bowel is not regularly emptied. Therefore, the first few years of life have to be supervised closely to make sure that all the necessary medication is given to stop the neorectum from becoming overfull, distended, and ectatic. While this problem is common to all forms of surgery for Hirschsprung's disease, fecal retention in the anterior pouch of a Duhamel procedure can be marked and a very long-term problem with late recurrences.

Fecal incontinence is also a long-term problem after surgery for Hirschsprung's disease. The incontinence may well precipitated by the lack of internal sphincter tone which is a deliberate part of the definitive procedure. If the sphincter is left intact, then enterocolitis and inability to empty in the first years of life are more likely, but if the sphincter is destroyed or partly destroyed by the surgery, then incontinence is more likely as a teenager.

In addition, where the fecal stream has been diverted before the surgery with a stoma, the peri-anal skin appears to be particularly sensitive to local excoriation after bowel continuity is restored. This can be so severe that defecation is very painful, and the surrounding skin can become badly scarred. This excoriation is common to both Hirschsprung's disease and to anorectal malformations where there has been a diverting colostomy prior to surgery.

**Major Complications**

Serious complications include **anastomotic leakage, spontaneous perforation, abscess formation,** and **abdominal sepsis,** which may lead to **systemic sepsis, multisystem organ failure** and even **death. Stricture formation** is not uncommon and may require repeated dilatations. **Repeated further surgery,** with or without stricture, may occur. **Bleeding** intra- and postoperatively can occur. **Fistula formation** may arise. **Fecal incontinence** and/or **fecal impaction** may occur, as can **anal skin excoriation** and the need for a **diverting stoma**. Where used **stomal problems** may arise and be considerable, even requiring further surgery or reversal.

# Surgery for Imperforate Anus and Anorectal Malformations

## Description

The anal canal is formed from fusion of the skin ectoderm and hindgut endoderm, where they have been separated by the perineal membrane. Failure to do this properly produces the various forms of imperforate anus, perhaps better described as anorectal malformation(s). Developmental fistulae to the perineum, bladder, and urethra occur in the male and to the vagina in the female. In an extreme form in the female, there is a common channel draining the urinary bladder and the hindgut – the cloaca – which can be 1–10 cm in length. Significant anorectal malformations occur in approximately 1:5,000 live births. Minor forms are more frequent but not well documented. They vary considerably from a stenosed opening to apparent absence of the anus. Essentially the anomalies are divided into *high* and *low* lesions. Some surgeons include an *intermediate* category also.

In *high* lesions, the hindgut ends above the sphincter complex and in the male is usually accompanied by a high fistula leading into the urethra or bladder. In the female with a high lesion, any fistula leads into the introitus of the vagina. There are also very complex anomalies that can produce a single channel, the cloaca, with or without duplication of the urogenital tract, and exstrophy of part or all of the urogenital and hindgut systems. A true rectal atresia is rare and appears to be a vascular accident in the already formed rectum. Rectal agenesis is relatively rare and usually occurs in patients with trisomy 21, where the bowel ends in the middle of the sphincters with no fistula. This is now included as an anorectal malformation.

In the *low* lesions, the bowel ends below the sphincter complex, and the end may be covered by skin in the male or comes to the surface as a subcutaneous fistula that travels forward to a varying degree. In the female, the low lesion is represented by an anterior ectopic anus, which is often stenosed, or a small opening in the introitus to the vagina.

Important associated anomalies include genitourinary defects, which occur in approximately 50 % of all patients with anorectal malformations. Associations with other anomalies or genetic problems include VACTERL (vertebral anomalies, anal atresia, cardiac malformations, tracheoesophageal fistula, renal anomalies, and limb anomalies), MURCS (Mullerian duct aplasia, renal aplasia, and cervicothoracic somite dysplasia), OEIS (omphalocele, exstrophy, imperforate anus, and spinal defects), trisomy 21, trisomy 13, trisomy 18, or Hirschsprung's disease.

In males, some 90 % patients require a posterior sagittal approach alone, while in 10 % an abdominal component (with laparotomy or laparoscopically) is necessary to mobilize a very high rectum. However, in females, in some 30 % of cloacas, the rectum or vagina is so high that an abdominal approach is needed (Khong et al. 1994).

### Anatomical Points

The anal canal is formed from fusion of the skin ectoderm and hindgut endoderm, and failure produces the various forms of imperforate anus and anorectal agenesis.

**Table 3.12** Surgery for imperforate anus/rectal agenesis estimated frequency of complications, risks, and consequences

| Complications, risks, and consequences | Estimated frequency |
|---|---|
| *Most significant/serious complications* | |
| Infection[a] | 5–20 % |
|   Subcutaneous | 5–20 % |
|   Intra-abdominal/pelvic (peritonitis; abscess) (especially in the ELBW; premature) | 5–20 % |
|   Systemic sepsis (especially in the ELBW; premature) | 2–5 % |
|   Hepatic portal sepsis (rare) | <0.1 % |
| Bleeding/hematoma formation[a] | |
|   Wound | 1–5 % |
|   Intra-abdominal | 0.1–1 % |
| Constipation[a] | 50–80 % |
| Fecal incontinence and fecalomas retention[a,b] | 20–50 % |
| Urinary incontinence[a,b] | 20–50 % |
| Recurrent fistula(e)[a,b] | 5–20 % |
| Stricture formation (anorectal)[a,b] | 5–20 % |
| Peri-anal excoriation[a,b] | 20–50 % |
| If an <u>abdominal component of surgery</u> is used | |
| Small bowel obstruction (postoperative early or late)[a] [Adhesion formation] | 1–5 % |
| Stomal problems[a] (prolapse; intussusception) | 5–20 % |
| Incisional hernia[a] | 5–20 % |
| *Rare significant/serious problems* | |
| Anastomotic leakage[a] | 0.1–1 % |
| Bowel injury (operative serious)[a] | 0.1–1 % |
| Ureteric injury (very rare)[a] | <0.1 % |
| Wound breakdown[a] | 0.1–1 % |
| Mortality <u>without</u> surgery (should surgery be refused)[a] | 50–80 % |
| *Less serious complications* | |
| Pain/tenderness | |
|   Acute (<4 weeks) | 5–20 % |
|   Chronic (>4 weeks) | <0.1 % |
| Paralytic ileus (peritonitis from preoperative perforation) | 20–30 % |
| Nerve parasthesia | 0.1–1 % |
| Wound scarring (poor cosmesis/wound deformity)[a] | 1–5 % |

[a]Dependent on underlying pathology, anatomy, surgical technique, and preferences
[b]Higher in patients with a common cloaca >3 cm
Note: ELBW extremely low-birth-weight newborn, <1,000 g
Important Note: Many of these complications are individually closely determined by the exact nature of the problem and surgery. The extent and underlying disease will alter the relative risks

Developmental fistulae are often present if minimal or no opening exists, and these will often complicate the surgery. True rectal atresia occurs in about 1 % of all cases of anorectal malformations.

## Perspective

See Table 3.12.


## Complications of the Anomaly

Anorectal malformations are often accompanied by other anomalies as noted, as it forms one of the anomalies that make up the VATER (or VACTERL) association. This includes congenital heart disease, tracheoesophageal fistulae, and renal disease as well as the anorectal malformation. Therefore, as the other lesions could be lethal, they greatly influence the outcome. At birth, intestinal obstruction will supervene in males with high and low lesions (where the lower part of the canal is a small caliber fistula, or the anus is covered with skin). In the female, intestinal obstruction is less common as even the high lesions have a fistula that ends in the introitus or vagina and allows for decompression.


## Complications of the Surgery

The level at which the bowel ends (with or without a continuing fistula) dictates the type of surgery. A *low anomaly* where the bowel passes through the sphincters before becoming a fistula requires a local procedure only: the anoplasty. A high lesion where the bowel ends above the sphincters before becoming a fistula requires more complex surgery, which can be done as a primary procedure in the neonate or after a temporary colostomy. The procedure is an anorectoplasty, a type of rectal pull-through reconstruction. As with Hirschsprung's disease, the surgical procedures and especially their timing are changing dramatically. Classical teaching is that for a low lesion, a cutback in either the male or female will suffice. While that may be true in the male, in the female this leaves a scarred perineum with the anterior lip of the anal canal still in the introitus. So, in the female, an anterior sagittal anorectoplasty is used either as a primary procedure after dilating the fistula up to a good size or after a temporary colostomy. In the high lesions in the male, a colostomy can be used while other investigations are carried out, but a primary procedure without a colostomy is now gaining popularity.

For *high lesions*, the classical treatment was a colostomy succeeded by investigations (to determine the actual level, connections to the urinary tract, etc.). Contrast studies through the stoma (if used) and up through the vagina in the female and through the urethra in both genders also help to define the anatomy before definitive surgery. Further investigations, e.g., an MRI to determine as accurately as possible the muscle anatomy (often grossly deficient in high lesions), will help with dissection and prognosis. In addition, the MRI may identify intraspinal lesions that may be the cause of the field defect in the first place. Furthermore, these spinal cord lesions may well contribute to poor sensation in the pelvis, in turn contributing to fecal and urinary incontinence and dysfunction.

**Major Complications**

Serious complications are less common with *low* anomalies, but include **infection, bleeding, abscess formation, anal stricture formation, fistula formation, wound breakdown, fecal impaction, constipation, and fecal incontinence** and **anal skin excoriation**. In *higher* lesions, these also occur, but additionally, where abdominal surgery is required, **anastomotic leakage, spontaneous perforation, abscess formation,** and **abdominal sepsis** may rarely lead to **systemic sepsis, multisystem organ failure,** and even **death**. **Repeated further surgery**, with or without stricture, may occur. **Incisional hernia** is reported. The need for a **diverting stoma**, where used may give rise to **stomal problems**, even requiring further surgery, or later reversal.

**Consent and Risk Reduction**

**Main Points to Explain**

- GA risk
- Pain/discomfort
- Bleeding/hematoma*
- Infection (local/systemic)*
- Feeding problems
- Nutritional deficiency
- Risk of other abdominal organ injury*
- Possible stoma
- Possible further surgery*
- Risks without surgery*
- Multisystem organ failure
- Death*

  **\*Dependent on pathology, comorbidities, and surgery performed**

# Surgery for Meckel's Diverticulum and Vitellointestinal Remnants

### Description

General anesthesia is used. The patient is usually positioned supine. The objective of the operation is to define the Meckel's diverticulum on the antimesenteric border and resect either the diverticulum itself or a section of the small bowel. If perforation has occurred, then drainage of purulent material and/or an abscess and peritoneal washout is necessary. The site of pain may "migrate" as the small bowel moves around in the abdominal cavity, making diagnosis more difficult. When an inverted Meckel's acts as the lead point for an intussusception, resection is necessary with primary anastomosis, but a stoma may be required if there is doubtful viability

+/− peritonitis. A good arterial blood supply in both bowel ends is essential before attempting an anastomosis. A single-layer interrupted technique using absorbable suture material is usually used by pediatric surgeons. In children, stapling techniques are rarely used.

The inspissated mucus of cystic fibrosis may act as a lead point, and the history of this disease should be sought. The disease increases the risks of complications (e.g., inspissated mucous obstruction and paralytic ileus after the procedure) including mortality risk. A patch of mucosa at the umbilicus requires simple excision; otherwise, it will persist, weeping mucus or bleeding. At excision (under a GA), care must be taken to look for a continuation deep into the abdominal cavity. A completely patent vitellointestinal duct is resected down to the true small bowel, through the umbilicus itself, or by minimal enlargement of the cicatrix. If there is a volvulus, it is reduced, and resection may be necessary.

## Anatomical Points

The communication between the small bowel and the yolk sac is usually completely obliterated and disappears before birth; however, in approximately 2–5 % of individuals, the communication may persist. A Meckel's diverticulum is one of the remnants of this vitellointestinal duct that connected the apex of the embryological midgut to the yolk sac. The duct can rarely be complete with an intestinal lumen from the ileum to the umbilicus, can be a complete band, can be part of a band with or without cysts in it, can be a Meckel's diverticulum, or can be any combinations of these. A band can serve as a point for volvulus of the small bowel. Rarely, the patent vitellointestinal duct may be associated with umbilical discharge. A Meckel's diverticulum may become inflamed, contain ectopic gastric or pancreatic mucosa, and bleed, obstruct, or ulcerate and perforate (in descending order of frequency). An island of pancreatic mucosa may be found in the intestinal wall without an accompanying diverticulum. The most common remnant, however, is a patch of mucosa in the umbilicus that persists after birth as a "felt-like" granuloma.

The diverticulum is often defined by the "rule of twos," within 2 ft (0.6 m) of the ileocecal valve (but can occur up to the jejunum), 2 in. (5 cm) long, 2 % population, and 2 % become complicated.

## Complications of the Anomaly

If the communication is completely patent as the vitellointestinal duct between the bowel and umbilicus, it will then discharge feces soon after birth. A Meckel's can act as the lead point for an intussusception. In this case the lead point can be a simple diverticulum, or the lead point can be a solid island of pancreatic mucosa (where there is no obvious diverticulum). There can be peptic ulceration and hemorrhage at the neck of the Meckel's when gastric mucosa is present. The hemorrhage may be sufficient to produce hypovolemia with marked bleeding PR. A

**Table 3.13** Surgery for Meckel's diverticulum and vitellointestinal remnants estimated frequency of complications, risks, and consequences

| Complications, risks, and consequences | Estimated frequency |
|---|---|
| *Most significant/serious complications* | |
| Infection[a] | 1–5 % |
| Subcutaneous | 1–5 % |
| Intra-abdominal/pelvic (peritonitis; abscess) (especially in the ELBW; premature) | 1–5 % |
| Systemic sepsis (especially in the ELBW; premature) | 1–5 % |
| Hepatic portal sepsis (rare) | <0.1 % |
| Bleeding/hematoma formation[a] | |
| Wound | 1–5 % |
| Intra-abdominal | 0.1–1 % |
| Small bowel obstruction (postoperative early or late)[a] [Adhesion formation] | 1–5 % |
| *Rare significant/serious problems* | |
| Anastomotic leakage[a] | 0.1–1 % |
| Bowel injury (operative serious)[a] | 0.1–1 % |
| Mortality | <0.1 % |
| *Less serious complications* | |
| Pain/tenderness | |
| Acute (<4 weeks) | 5–20 % |
| Chronic (>4 weeks) | <0.1 % |
| Paralytic ileus (peritonitis from preoperative perforation) | 20–30 % |
| Wound scarring (poor cosmesis/wound deformity)[a] | 1–5 % |

[a]Dependent on underlying pathology, anatomy, surgical technique, and preferences
Note: ELBW extremely low-birth-weight newborn, <1,000 g
Important Note: Many of these complications are individually closely determined by the exact nature of the problem and surgery. The extent and underlying disease will alter the relative risks

simple Meckel's itself can give rise to local inflammation and peritonitis similar to appendicitis, especially where the Meckel's is narrow necked. Cysts in the remnant can be in the abdominal wall, where they can give rise to repeated infections and discharge through the umbilicus. Where there is a band from the abdominal wall to point of attachment to the intestine, segmental volvulus can occur around this band.

## Perspective

See Table 3.13. The complications of any of these procedures will depend on the initial pathology encountered. Where there is bowel obstruction, preoperative perforation and sepsis increase the risk of postoperative complications, the most serious complication being anastomotic leakage, the risk of which is increased by distal obstruction of any cause. It is therefore vital to alleviate any significant obstruction distal to level of anastomosis (but this is highly unlikely with a Meckel's). The consequence of an anastomotic leakage is contamination of the peritoneal cavity leading to generalized peritonitis or intra-abdominal abscess formation, typically in the paracolic gutters, pelvis, or the subphrenic spaces. The incidence of anastomotic leakages is reduced by ensuring good blood supply to the bowel ends, minimal tension, and no factors contraindicating an anastomosis. Wound infection, small bowel obstruction, and enterocutaneous fistula are significant, but fortunately uncommon complications.

## Major Complications

Where there is bowel obstruction, preoperative perforation and sepsis increase the risk of postoperative complications. The most serious complication is **anastomotic leakage**. But, this is uncommon in the young patient. **Wound infection, small bowel obstruction,** and **enterocutaneous fistula** are significant, but fortunately uncommon complications. **Systemic sepsis** is uncommon, but is increased when delayed diagnosis occurs, and is rarely followed by multisystem organ failure and even death.

---

**Consent and Risk Reduction**

**Main Points to Explain**

- GA risk
- Pain/discomfort
- Bleeding/hematoma*
- Infection (local/systemic)*
- Risk of other abdominal organ injury*
- Possible stoma
- Possible further surgery*
- Risks without surgery*
- Multisystem organ failure
- Death*

**\*Dependent on pathology, comorbidities, and surgery performed**

---

# Surgery for Intussusception

## Description

General anesthesia is used. The patient is positioned supine. The objective of the operation is to define the problem and alleviate the obstruction. Resection of bowel may be required depending on the pathology and degree of fixity, obstruction, ischemia, or necrosis present. For children, a transverse muscle-cutting incision is typically used.

**Intussusception** is an invagination (telescoping) of proximal bowel into distal bowel, eventually causing obstruction. This is not a common disease in the newborn, but is a common disease in infants from 6 to 10 months of age, and after that, the disease gradually becomes less common again. It is temporally related to the time of weaning, the introduction of non-sterile foods, and the seasons when viral infection (and possibly localized swelling of Peyer's patches) is more common (spring and autumn). The usual form is an invagination of the terminal ileum and ileocecal junction into the ascending colon. It is the most frequent cause of intestinal obstruction in the first 2 years of life. Some 75–90 % of cases can be reduced by using a form of hydrostatic enema (barium, air, or saline), under imaging control.

Over the years, that has progressed from a barium enema to an air enema, to ultrasound (U/S) diagnosis (far more accurate than a plain X-ray) with ultrasound-controlled reduction using a saline enema. The latter avoids all radiation (some 70 % of barium enemas ordered for suspected intussusception showed that there was none) and avoids risk of perforation and barium peritonitis. Surgery may be required if hydrostatic pressure reduction is unsuccessful or, for multiple recurrences, as either an open or a laparoscopic procedure, with the occasional patient requiring bowel resection for ischemia, or more rarely because there is a small bowel tumor (6 % chance in the older age groups, and usually a lymphoma).

## Anatomical Points

There are few real anatomical aspects that are pertinent to intussusception, except for the presence of a Meckel's diverticulum, swollen Peyer's patches, or bowel tumor mass which can all act as a firm leading bolus which can then be moved down the gut with peristaltic contractions.

## Complications of the Lesion

Intussusception will progressively involve more and more of the bowel as it telescopes. This leads to a bowel obstruction and to progressive loss of blood supply. Eventually there will be a venous gangrene of the intussusceptum. Once that has become established, bowel resection is inevitable. If the intussusception still has not been treated, then bacteremia and endotoxic shock can ensue.

## Complications of Nonsurgical Intervention (Radiology)

Hydrostatic or pneumostatic reduction using an enema (with imaging) can lead to a perforation of the weakened bowel as pressure is applied. The combination of barium and feces in the peritoneal cavity is potentially lethal, so that other modalities have been sought. The first was to use air with an image intensifier, then saline reduction using U/S. The last has the advantages of being able to diagnose the lesion (before the enema) and to effect a treatment, both without radiation.

**Table 3.14** Surgery for intussusception estimated frequency of complications, risks, and consequences

| Complications, risks, and consequences | Estimated frequency |
|---|---|
| *Most significant/serious complications* | |
| Infection[a] | 1–5 % |
|   Subcutaneous | 1–5 % |
|   Intra-abdominal/pelvic (peritonitis; abscess) (especially in the ELBW; premature) | 1–5 % |
|   Systemic sepsis (especially in the ELBW; premature) | 1–5 % |
|   Hepatic portal sepsis (rare) | <0.1 % |
| Bleeding/hematoma formation[a] | |
|   Wound | 1–5 % |
|   Intra-abdominal | 0.1–1 % |
| Small bowel obstruction (postoperative early or late)[a] [Adhesion formation] | 1–5 % |
| Recurrent intussusception[a] | 5–20 % |
| *Rare significant/serious problems* | |
| Perforation[b] (spontaneous preoperative) | 0.1–1 % |
| Anastomotic leakage[a] (when performed) | 0.1–1 % |
| Bowel injury (operative serious)[a] | 0.1–1 % |
| Mortality | <0.1 % |
| *Less serious complications* | |
| Pain/tenderness | |
|   Acute (<4 weeks) | 5–20 % |
|   Chronic (>4 weeks) | <0.1 % |
| Paralytic ileus (peritonitis from preoperative perforation) | 20–30 % |
| Wound scarring (poor cosmesis/wound deformity)[a] | 1–5 % |

[a]Dependent on underlying pathology, anatomy, surgical technique, and preferences
[b]Spontaneous perforation may occur, as can perforation in association with hydraulic reduction techniques
Note: ELBW extremely low-birth-weight newborn, <1,000 g
Important Note: Many of these complications are individually closely determined by the exact nature of the problem and surgery. The extent and underlying disease will alter the relative risks

## Complications of Surgery

Failure to reduce the intussusception will lead to a bowel resection. But, in the more common ileo-ileocolic intussusception, reduction can often be achieved even after failure of radiological intervention. If a resection is still required, then there is the potential for stricturing at the site of the anastomosis if the ends of the intestine were still ischemic at the points of resection. More likely to cause a stricture, however, is where partially devitalized intestine is put back after reduction without resection.

## Recurrences

**Recurrences** after radiological or surgical reduction do occur, approximately 10 % after radiological reduction and approximately 5 % after surgical reduction. The first recurrence is treated in the same way as the first presentation with similar results. Repeated recurrences occur and are treated in a similar fashion. Individual surgeons have different thresholds for surgery to try to prevent repeated recurrences, and the surgery for the recurrences is not always successful. Carrying out a fixation of the cecum is now rarely used. A simple appendectomy diminishes the recurrence rate but not entirely; a right hemicolectomy is radical but is nearly always successful. But, just waiting through the multiple recurrences that can occur is as successful, but distressing to the family.

### Major Complications

See Table 3.14. Where there is bowel obstruction, preoperative perforation and sepsis increase the risk of postoperative complications. The most serious complication is **anastomotic leakage**. But, this is uncommon in the young patient. **Wound infection**, **small bowel obstruction**, and **enterocutaneous fistula** are significant, but fortunately uncommon complications. **Recurrent intussusception** can occur. **Small bowel obstruction** due to adhesions may occur at any stage. **Systemic sepsis** is uncommon, but is increased when delayed diagnosis occurs, and is rarely followed by multisystem organ failure and even death.

---

**Consent and Risk Reduction**

**Main Points to Explain**

- GA risk
- Pain/discomfort
- Bleeding/hematoma*
- Infection (local/systemic)*
- Risk of other abdominal organ injury*
- Possible stoma
- Possible further surgery*
- Risks without surgery*
- Multisystem organ failure
- Death*

   ***Dependent on pathology, comorbidities, and surgery performed**

---

# Pediatric Surgery in the Older Child

## *Introduction*

*Abdominal wall defects in the older child* are typically small umbilical herniae due to failure of a congenital defect to close completely after birth and on occasions may be larger and strangulate or obstruct. If these herniae fail to close by 2 years of age or are symptomatic, surgical repair is advisable. Surgery for inguinal herniae is performed in the newborn and infant in most situations, where early repair is advisable, but may also present in the older child and require surgical repair.

*General abdominal surgical procedures in the older child* include a variety of procedures principally related to inflammation, reflux, feeding access, or tumor.

Some of the surgical procedures described in section "Pediatric Surgery in the Newborn and Infant" may apply to surgery in the older child in certain situations, such as when diagnostic features are more subtle, for example, from incomplete lower-grade gut obstruction, which may present later.

# Abdominal Wall Defect Surgery

## Surgery for Umbilical/Supraumbilical/Epigastric Herniae

### Description

General anesthesia is used. Umbilical herniae (UH) are present in up to 85 % of premature newborns and approximately 20 % of full-term newborns. Over 90 % will close by the age of 2–5 years in Caucasians, but much later (teenagers) in Africans. Therefore, surgery should not be performed for simple umbilical herniae until after these ages, respectively, unless symptomatic. Supraumbilical herniae virtually never close on their own, so surgery can be carried out at the most suitable age for the child and the institution concerned (outside children's hospitals, many anesthetists are uneasy about GA use for children <3 years of age). Umbilical herniae are through the embryological physiological defect at the umbilical cord where the expanding midgut herniates, but then returns to the abdominal cavity by 10 weeks of gestation. Supraumbilical herniae are also congenital defects in the abdominal wall cicatrix just above the center of the umbilicus, then turning inferiorly. Paraumbilical hernial defects laterally to the umbilicus are extremely rare in children. In those over 2 years of age with central umbilical hernia and in those with a supraumbilical hernia, the surgery is essentially the same. A peritoneal sac is usually present containing omentum, or less commonly bowel, particularly in larger herniae. In obese children, the diagnosis may be especially difficult. Symptoms from an umbilical hernia are extremely rare in children; therefore, surgery is essentially for cosmetic reasons alone. Incarceration and bowel obstruction are almost unheard of in children but would require emergency intervention. A transverse skin incision is made below the umbilicus. The sac is defined and excised at the edge of the linea defect and from the overlying skin of the umbilicus. The contents are reduced, and the defect is closed as an overlapping two-layer closure (Mayo) with heavy absorbable sutures or as a two-layer turned-in (Keel) repair. Mesh is sometimes used.

**Table 3.15** Surgery for umbilical/supraumbilical/epigastric herniae in the older child estimated frequency of complications, risks, and consequences

| Complications, risks, and consequences | Estimated frequency |
|---|---|
| *Most significant/serious complications* | |
| Infection | 1–5 % |
| Hernia recurrence[a] (10 year) | 0.1–1 % |
| Suture abscess +/– suture sinus[a] | 0.1–1 % |
| Bleeding (including intra-abdominal) | <0.1 % |
| *Less serious complications* | |
| Pain/discomfort/tenderness | |
| (<2 months; days only in children) | 20–50 % |
| Pain/discomfort/tenderness | |
| (>2 months) | 0.1–1 % |
| Bruising or hematoma formation[a] | 5–20 % |
| Dimpling/deformity of the skin[a] | 1–5 % |
| Scarring | 1–5 % |

[a]Dependent on underlying pathology, anatomy, hernia type, surgical technique, and preferences

Epigastric herniae are midline defects in the linea alba anywhere between the umbilicus and the xiphoid. Because the falciform ligament and its fat are deep to these defects, they never contain viscera. They rarely cause symptoms, but the free edge of the defect may nip the herniated fat to cause very localized pain. If that happens, then it is worthwhile closing the defect with absorbable sutures; otherwise, it is again a cosmetic issue. These can be seen in the child, but effectively disappear in the adult as the subcutaneous fat becomes thicker.

### Anatomical Points

The main variance is in the site of the hernia as described above, and extreme versions of each, which are exceedingly rare. Multiple defects are also extremely rare.

### Perspective

See Table 3.15. The complications related to UH, SUH, and epigastric hernia repair are generally minimal. Local bruising and superficial wound infection may occur.

### Major Complications

**Infection** from skin, and occasionally bowel organisms, may occur. **Bleeding** is seldom severe, often from omental or mesenteric vessels, and may increase risk of infection. Established infection may rarely necessitate **removal of mesh or sutures**.

**Hernia recurrence** is uncommon and further increased with obesity.

---

**Consent and Risk Reduction**

**Main Points to Explain**

- GA risk
- Pain/discomfort
- Bleeding/hematoma*
- Infection (local/systemic)*
- Risk of other abdominal organ injury*
- Hernia recurrence
- Possible further surgery*
- Risks without surgery*

**\*Dependent on pathology, comorbidities, and surgery performed**

---

# *General Abdominal Surgery*

## Open Gastrostomy

### Description

General anesthesia is used. The aim is to establish a portal to the stomach from the exterior so as to be able to feed the child. A small RUQ transverse incision is made over the stomach at a position where the gastrostomy will not impinge on the rib cage (as the child grows, the skin migrates upward). At open surgery, a button device (a short, valved feeding tube that has a small flat external flange which sits flush on the skin) is usually inserted directly into the stomach and held in place with two purse-string sutures. The stomach is also sutured to the anterior abdominal wall, with at least three sutures. Occasionally an 18 G Foley catheter may be used rather than a button. The abdomen is then closed around the gastrostomy. Some surgeons will bring the gastrostomy out through a separate stab wound.

### Anatomical Points

The colon, small bowel, liver, and omentum may overlie the stomach and make access difficult. Although these organs are at risk, generally these can be displaced easily in children to enable the procedure to be performed. Patients with cerebral palsy often have curved spines that will occasionally prevent the stomach being brought to the anterior abdominal wall. Then, an alternative procedure will have to be found (e.g., a feeding jejunostomy).

**Table 3.16** Open gastrostomy estimated frequency of complications, risks, and consequences

| Complications, risks, and consequences | Estimated frequency |
|---|---|
| *Most significant/serious complications* | |
| Infection | |
|   Wound granulation around the button/catheter | 5–20 % |
|   Subcutaneous cellulitis; abscess | 1–5 % |
|   Intraperitoneal leak | 1–5 % |
|   Systemic[a] | 0.1–1 % |
| Bleeding/hematoma formation | 1–5 % |
| Gastric leakage[a] | 5–10 % |
| Gastrocutaneous fistula (persistent after removal) | 1–5 % |
| Aspiration pneumonitis | |
|   Overall | 1–5 % |
|   In those with CNS defects | 5–20 % |
| *Less serious complications* | |
| Discharging abscess sinus | 1–5 % |
| Incisional hernia formation | 0.1–1 % |
| Tube dislodgment (internalization or extraction) | 5–20 % |
| Gastroesophageal reflux[a] | 5–20 % |
| Paralytic ileus | 1–5 % |
| Scarring/wound deformity | 5–20 % |

[a]Dependent on underlying pathology, anatomy, surgical technique, and preferences

## Perspective

See Table 3.16. Pediatric gastrostomy is used for feeding and very rarely for drainage. Gastrostomy feeding is especially important for patients who are unable to feed or spill into their lungs on feeding. The most common type of patient will have brain damage, e.g., patients with cerebral palsy. The procedure is often combined with a fundoplication, as a gastrostomy will usually increase any reflux that is present or may cause reflux de novo. Some 5–20 % of patients will get reflux for the first time, and others will experience deterioration of any reflux already present. Where possible a percutaneous endoscopic gastrostomy (PEG) is used, so that an open procedure is avoided. Recently laparoscopic gastrostomy has been introduced using increasing sizes of dilator introduced under laparoscopic control and over a guide wire. This is especially useful in those who have undergone a fundoplication as part of the same procedure.

## Major Complications

If a Foley catheter is used as the first access device (rather than a button), the balloon of the Foley catheter may occasionally migrate distally and can lead to **stomach outlet obstruction**. Therefore, buttons are now more commonly used as the initial device after open fundoplication in children, as being so short they cannot migrate. Separation of the stomach from the anterior abdominal wall may result in **intraperitoneal**

**leakage** of stomach contents and peritonitis, with or without abscess formation or generalized sepsis. This is most likely to occur at the first change of a button or catheter. If the new button or catheter is pushed down the track blind, the stomach can be pushed off the abdominal wall. Therefore, in pediatric practice, the first change is often covered by an upper GI endoscopy to make sure that the new device is in place. **Pressure necrosis** of the stomach against the catheter balloon and free **perforation** is rare. The most frequent complication, however, occurs around the exit of the catheter where **minor infection** and exuberant **granulation tissue** form. **Gastric acid leaks around the tube** may cause **excoriation.** Associated **abscess formation** is uncommon. **Systemic sepsis** is rare, but may be severe, often related to the underlying condition(s), and can lead to death. Persistent **gastrocutaneous fistula** after removal of the device is not uncommon after prolonged use of a gastrostomy and infrequently can be persistent, but most close. **Aspiration pneumonitis** may occur in any patient, but risk in those with cerebral palsy and other CNS lesions may be as high as 20 %.

---

**Consent and Risk Reduction**

**Main Points to Explain**

- GA risk
- Pain/discomfort
- Bleeding/hematoma*
- Infection (local/systemic)*
- Risk of other abdominal organ injury*
- Intraperitoneal leakage
- Leakage around tube
- Skin excoriation
- Migration and pyloric obstruction
- Possible further surgery*
- Risks without surgery*

   ***Dependent on pathology, comorbidities, and surgery performed**

---

# Percutaneous Endoscopic Gastrostomy

## Description

In children, general anesthesia is used for percutaneous endoscopic gastrostomy (PEG). The aim is to establish a portal to the stomach from the exterior. The peroral endoscope is turned anteriorly inside the stomach so that the scope light is visible through the anterior abdominal wall. The surgeon placing the PEG indents the stomach at the best point to place a gastrostomy. A small stab incision is made through the skin only, and a trocar and cannula (in the PEG set) is inserted into the stomach under endoscopic control. A flexible looped wire is inserted through this into the stomach and grasped by the endoscopist and pulled out with the endoscope through the mouth. The PEG catheter (usually 18FG has a pointed tip with a guide wire and a flange at the rear end) is then tied to the wire and pulled back point first through the stomach and abdominal wall. The flange at the back end of the catheter pulls the stomach wall up against the abdominal wall. There are no stitches so tension has to be maintained by using a tightly fitting external flange. This catheter will be replaced by a button 6 weeks to 3 months later, under endoscopic control. The stomach wall is usually adherent to the abdominal wall by then, thereby avoiding leakage of feeds into the peritoneal cavity, although this can occur at any time, should the stomach and abdominal wall separate.

**Anatomical Points**

The colon, small bowel, liver, and omentum may overlie the stomach, and as the stomach is inflated by the gastroenterologist to get visualization, the greater curvature of the stomach tends to rotate upward pulling the colon and small bowel in front. As a result, the trocar and cannula may then go through one of those before getting into the stomach. This can lead to the PEG being gradually pulled through the stomach wall over time and dislodging into that organ (colon or small bowel). Once that has occurred, it will produce marked diarrhea. Obesity or curvature of the spine may also make the procedure more challenging.

**Perspective**

See Table 3.17. Gastrostomy is used for feeding in children. Percutaneous endoscopic gastrostomy (PEG) is almost exclusively used for gastric access, where an endoscopy can be performed. Complications are few, but misplacement of the catheter through another viscus can occur, and skin infection and irritation are common. Change from the PEG catheter to a button has a sufficiently high risk of pushing the stomach away from the abdominal wall that endoscopy is now routinely used at this first change to make sure that the new device has travelled down the new track correctly and is now in the stomach. The risk of intraperitoneal feed leakage can be as high as 10 % if endoscopy is not used at the first changeover. The balloon and valved buttons frequently fail and have to be replaced. Endoscopy is not usually required after the first change, unless difficulties are encountered. Inability to perform the procedure can be as high as 10 % especially in the very young, those with a badly deformed spine and oro-esophageal problems, after prior upper GI surgery, and if the procedure is accompanied by a laparoscopic fundoplication. Aspiration pneumonitis may be as high as 20–30 % in those with CNS defects. Perforation of the colon or small bowel by the catheter during PEG insertion can be as high as 5–10 %, but can be reduced with proper illumination

**Table 3.17** Percutaneous endoscopic gastrostomy estimated frequency of complications, risks, and consequences

| Complications, risks, and consequences | Estimated frequency |
|---|---|
| *Most significant/serious complications* | |
| Infection | |
|    Wound granulations | 5–20 % |
|    Subcutaneous cellulitis; abscess | 1–5 % |
|    Intraperitoneal leak | 1–5 % |
|    Systemic | 0.1–1 % |
| Bleeding/hematoma formation[a] | 1–5 % |
| Gastric leakage into the peritoneal cavity[a] (higher risk at first changeover) | 1–5 % |
| Persistent gastric fistula (following removal) | 1–5 % |
| Discharging abscess sinus | 1–5 % |
| Free esophageal/gastric perforation | 1–5 % |
| Failure to perform endoscopically[a] | 5–20 % |
| Tube dislodgment (internalization or extraction) and duodenal obstruction | 5–20 % |
| Aspiration pneumonitis | |
|    Overall | 1–5 % |
|    In those with CNS defects | 5–20 % |
| Catheter going through colon or small bowel[a] | 1–5 % |
| Conversion to open laparotomy/laparoscopy[a] (early or late) | 0.1–1 % |
| *Less serious complications* | |
| Paralytic ileus | 1–5 % |
| Pneumoperitoneum | 5–20 % |
| Gas bloating (transient) | 5–20 % |
| Gastroesophageal reflux | 5–20 % |
| Injury to mouth, teeth, pharynx, or larynx | 1–5 % |
| Hernia formation (incisional) | 0.1–1 % |

[a]Dependent on underlying pathology, anatomy, surgical technique, and preferences

and extra care. Laparoscopic gastrostomy can now be employed which avoids the potential for an esophageal injury and also reduce risk of colonic or small bowel injury.

## Major Complications

Occasionally, the flange of the initial PEG catheter may migrate distally and can lead to **stomach outlet obstruction**. Separation of the stomach from the anterior abdominal wall will result in **intraperitoneal leakage** of stomach contents and **peritonitis**, with or without **abscess formation** or generalized **sepsis**. **Pressure necrosis** of the stomach against the catheter balloon and free **perforation** is very rare in children. The most frequent complication, however, occurs around the exit of the catheter where exuberant **granulation tissue** and **excoriation** from acid leakage are common. Associated **abscess formation** is not uncommon. **Systemic sepsis** is infrequent, but may be severe, often related to the underlying condition(s), and can lead to **death.** Although PEG approach is usually easy and safe, additional risks of **esophageal perforation** or **teeth injury** can occur, but are very infrequent. Persistent **gastrocutaneous fistula** is not uncommon after prolonged use of a gastrostomy and infrequently can be persistent, but most close.

**Consent and Risk Reduction**

**Main Points to Explain**

- GA risk
- Pain/discomfort
- Bleeding/hematoma*
- Infection (local/systemic)*
- Risk of other abdominal organ injury*
- Intraperitoneal leakage
- Leakage around tube
- Skin excoriation
- Migration and pyloric obstruction
- Possible further surgery*
- Risks without surgery*

*****Dependent on pathology, comorbidities, and surgery performed**

# Open Gastroesophageal (Nissen) Fundoplication

## Description

General anesthesia is used. The aim is to form a ring of stomach around the lower part of the esophagus, as a complete sleeve, by wrapping the upper fundus of the stomach from the left around behind the lower esophagus to bring it in front of the esophagus, to be sutured in front to the non-wrapped part of the fundus. In that way, it acts as a higher-pressure zone, allowing food and drink in, but not allowing either to reflux. There are many variations to this operation; however, the basic variations are:

1. Taking the anterolateral wall of the fundus of the stomach and sliding it up and around behind the esophagus and then sewing it to itself in front of the esophagus. This operation does not require division of the short gastric vessels.
2. Division of the short gastric vessels may be required if the spleen is pulled into the gap behind the stomach as the wrap is achieved. In pediatric patients, short gastric division is rarely required if the bands from the diaphragm to the esophagus and stomach are adequately divided – especially on the left side.

Most surgeons use a large bougie (30–36 FrG) within the esophageal lumen, while the wrap is being undertaken to try to prevent making the wrap too tight, but with experience, the bougie is often no longer required.

## Anatomical Points

Very infrequently the anterior wall of the stomach is not generous enough to be taken around behind the esophagus without division of the short gastric vessels. The short gastric vessels may be very high on the greater curvature of the stomach or tightly applied to the spleen. The abdominal esophagus may be very short. Adhesions to the spleen, diaphragm, or colon may exist. Liver or splenic enlargement may reduce access to the stomach. Rare anomalies of the vascular supply to the stomach may render the stomach fundus susceptible to ischemia upon division of the short gastric vessels, especially with tensioning of the stomach. There may be a hiatus hernia, which will have to be dealt with, and the extra care taken in the closure of the hiatus. Occasionally the stomach cannot be brought to the abdominal wall because of spinal curvature blocking the access (not uncommon in cerebral palsy patients).

## Perspective

See Table 3.18. Many types of fundoplication exist, and within the Nissen-type alone, controversy persists as to whether the short gastrics should or should not be divided in total fundoplications. The "physiological fundoplication" of Boix Ochoa uses a procedure that increases the angle of His and does an anterior wrap only suturing it to the right crus and then a hitch of the fundus to the left diaphragm. Partial fundoplications are variously described with the wrap only encircling the posterior 180°–270° of the esophagus, and similarly anterior partial fundoplications, encircling part of the anterior part of the esophagus. In those who are neurologically impaired, a partial fundoplication rarely works. They may, however, be appropriate for a second procedure in neurologically intact children, where the first fundoplication produced unrelenting dysphagia that has to be relieved surgically. Even then, they frequently fail. As the child grows, the wraps become looser, so that partial wraps are more likely to fail with time, and tight wraps will slacken, so that dysphagia relents. Open fundoplications have been largely replaced by laparoscopic approaches. Exceptions occur. The most common would be where there have been multiple abdominal procedures and adhesions; the most extreme would be where neither an open abdominal nor a laparoscopic procedure can be achieved. An example would be after an exomphalos major repair at birth, where the liver now overlies the stomach and is attached to the spleen with adhesions, making access to the upper stomach impossible through the abdomen alone, where a thoracoabdominal approach is often necessary. Dysphagia is frequent early but declines to 5–10 % by 6 months. Similarly, gas bloat syndrome is higher early on but improves over the

**Table 3.18** Open gastroesophageal (Nissen) fundoplication estimated frequency of complications, risks, and consequences

| Complications, risks, and consequences | Estimated frequency |
|---|---|
| **Most significant/serious complications** | |
| Infection[a] | |
|    Subcutaneous/wound | 1–5 % |
|    Intra-abdominal | 0.1–1 % |
|    Mediastinitis | <0.1 % |
|    Intrathoracic (pneumonia; pleural) | 1–5 % |
|    Subphrenic abscess | 0.1–1 % |
|    Systemic | 0.1–1 % |
|    Late – post-splenectomy sepsis (vaccination) | <0.1 % |
| Bleeding and hematoma formation[a] | 1–5 % |
| Dysphagia (>6 months postoperatively) | 5–20 % |
| Persistent or recurrent gastroesophageal reflux (lifetime) | 5–20 % |
| Gas bloat syndrome | |
|    (<6 months postoperatively) | 5–20 % |
|    (>6 months postoperatively) | 1–5 % |
| Inability to vomit or belch[a] | 5–20 % |
| Diaphragmatic injury | 1–5 % |
| Diaphragmatic (paraesophageal or wrap) herniation[a] | 5–20 % |
| Breakdown of fundoplication[a] | |
|    Overall | 1–5 % |
|    In the neurologically impaired | 20–50 % |
| Delayed gastric emptying[a] | 1–5 % |
| Bilious vomiting | 1–5 % |
| Dumping syndrome[a] | |
|    (>6 months postoperatively) | 1–5 % |
|    (<6 months postoperatively) | 5–20 % |
| Diarrhea | 5–20 % |
| Small bowel obstruction (early or late; lifetime risk)[a] [Adhesion formation] | 1–5 % |
| **Rare significant/serious problems** | |
| Liver injury[a] | 0.1–1 % |
| Splenic injury[a] (rarely splenectomy) | 0.1–1 % |
| Pancreatic injury/pancreatitis/pancreatic cyst/leakage/pancreatic fistula | 0.1–1 % |
| Bowel injury (duodenum, small bowel, colon)[a] | 0.1–1 % |
| Pneumothorax | 0.1–1 % |
| Death[a] | <0.1 % |
| **Less serious complications** | |
| Paralytic ileus | 1–5 % |
| Intolerance of large meals (necessity for small frequent meals) | 50–80 % |
| Excessive flatus[a] | 50–80 % |
| Pain/tenderness | |
|    Acute (<4 weeks) | 5–20 % |
|    Chronic (>4 weeks) | <0.1 % |
| Wound scarring (poor cosmesis/wound deformity) | 1–5 % |
| Incisional hernia | 0.1–1 % |
| Nasogastric tube[a] | 50–80 % |

[a]Dependent on underlying pathology, anatomy, surgical technique, and preferences

years. Inability to vomit or belch is much higher in the pediatric population, but is diminishing as the wraps are now shorter and looser. Dysphagia, gas bloat syndrome, and inability to vomit or belch reflect a too tight wrap. Persistent gastroesophageal reflux in pediatrics, which reflects failure or excessive looseness of the wrap, is ~5–10 % for otherwise normal children, but as high as 30–50 % in neurologically impaired children.

The incidence of hiatus hernia, including or excluding the wrap, is high in children where (in days gone by) the hiatus was not closed behind the esophagus. There is probably a 15 % increased lifetime risk of hiatus hernia, and this could be as high as 20 % in the first 5 years in those who are neurologically impaired, but again closing the hiatus has reduced this substantially. Breakdown of the fundoplication occurs in ~1–5 % of cases overall, but up to 50 % in neurologically impaired patients. Similarly, delayed gastric emptying occurs in ~1–5 % of cases, but increases to ~20 % of neurologically impaired patients.

## Major Complications

The most common major complication is **aphagia**, or very severe **dysphagia**, which can occasionally require very **early reoperation** (within days). **Persistent or recurrent gastroesophageal reflux** can occur after failure of the surgery either initially or later, with loosening of the wrap. Damage to the spleen that requires **splenectomy** is very rare in children. Full-thickness **esophageal or gastric** damage is a major complication, but this occurs very infrequently indeed; in primary anti-reflux surgery, it is usually seen immediately and repaired immediately. **Infection and multisystem failure** are very rare, but a late perforation or undetected leak can occur to cause this. **Bleeding** is rare and is usually controlled at surgery.

**Consent and Risk Reduction**

**Main Points to Explain**

- GA risk
- Pain/discomfort
- Bleeding/hematoma*
- Infection (local/systemic)*
- Risk of other abdominal organ injury*
- Intraperitoneal leakage
- Dysphagia
- Recurrence of reflux
- Possible further surgery*
- Risks without surgery*

**\*Dependent on pathology, comorbidities, and surgery performed**

# Laparoscopic Gastroesophageal (Nissen) Fundoplication

## Description

General anesthesia is used. The aim of the procedure is the production of a one-way valve between the esophagus and stomach and is identical to that for open fundoplication. Most surgeons use five ports in this procedure, although the epigastric port used for retraction is sometimes replaced with the Nathanson hook retractor. In pediatric patients, division of the short gastric vessels is rarely required. The mobilization of the anterior wall of the stomach and the esophagus is similar to that carried out in open fundoplication with the exception that dissection behind the esophagus and exposure of the pillars of the hiatus are more frequently carried out during laparoscopic fundoplication. This is because it is necessary to create a clear window behind the esophagus to safely and more easily draw the stomach through behind the esophagus. For this reason almost all surgeons today practice narrowing of the hiatus posteriorly with one, two, or more sutures.

## Anatomical Points

The chief variation which has practical importance in laparoscopic fundoplication relates to the size of the left lobe of the liver. When this is large and bulky, it can obscure vision of the hiatus. Previous surgery can be problematic, altering anatomy. Very rarely, abnormal blood supply of the stomach fundus may cause ischemia, especially after short gastric vessel division.

**Table 3.19** Laparoscopic gastroesophageal (Nissen) fundoplication estimated frequency of complications, risks, and consequences

| Complications, risks, and consequences | Estimated frequency |
| --- | --- |
| *Most significant/serious complications* | |
| Infection[a] | |
|    Subcutaneous/wound | 1–5 % |
|    Intra-abdominal | 0.1–1 % |
|    Mediastinitis | <0.1 % |
|    Intrathoracic (pneumonia; pleural) | 1–5 % |
|    Subphrenic abscess | 0.1–1 % |
|    Systemic | 0.1–1 % |
|    Late – post-splenectomy sepsis (vaccination) | <0.1 % |
| Bleeding or hematoma formation[a] | 1–5 % |
| Dysphagia (>6 months postoperatively) | 5–20 % |
| Persistent or recurrent gastroesophageal reflux (lifetime) | 5–20 % |
| Gas bloat syndrome | |
|    (<6 months postoperatively) | 5–20 % |
|    (>6 months postoperatively) | 1–5 % |

**Table 3.19** (continued)

| Complications, risks, and consequences | Estimated frequency |
| --- | --- |
| Inability to vomit or belch[a] | 5–20 % |
| Conversion to open operation | 1–5 % |
| Diaphragmatic injury | 1–5 % |
| Diaphragmatic (paraesophageal or wrap) herniation[a] | 5–20 % |
| Breakdown of fundoplication[a] | |
| Overall | 1–5 % |
| In the neurologically impaired | 20–50 % |
| Delayed gastric emptying | 1–5 % |
| Bilious vomiting | 1–5 % |
| Dumping syndrome | |
| (>6 months postoperatively) | 1–5 % |
| (<6 months postoperatively) | 5–20 % |
| Diarrhea | 5–20 % |
| Small bowel obstruction (early or late; lifetime risk)[a] [Adhesion formation] | 1–5 % |
| *Rare significant/serious problems* | |
| Splenic injury[a] (rarely splenectomy) | 0.1–1 % |
| Pancreatic injury/pancreatitis/pancreatic cyst/leakage/pancreatic fistula | 0.1–1 % |
| Bowel injury (duodenum, small bowel, colon) | 0.1–1 % |
| Liver injury | 0.1–1 % |
| Pneumothorax | 0.1–1 % |
| Gas embolus | 0.1–1 % |
| *Less serious complications* | |
| Paralytic ileus | 1–5 % |
| Intolerance of large meals (necessity for small frequent meals) | 50–80 % |
| Excessive flatus[a] | 50–80 % |
| Surgical emphysema | 1–5 % |
| Pain/tenderness | |
| Acute (<4 weeks) | 5–20 % |
| Chronic (>4 weeks) | <0.1 % |
| Wound scarring (poor cosmesis/wound deformity) | 1–5 % |
| Port-site herniae | 0.1–1 % |
| Incisional hernia | 0.1–1 % |
| Nasogastric tube[a] | 50–80 % |

[a]Dependent on underlying pathology, anatomy, surgical technique, and preferences

## Perspective

See Table 3.19. Many types of fundoplication exist, and within the Nissen-type alone, controversy persists as to whether the short gastrics should or should not be divided in total fundoplications, but in pediatric surgery, short gastric division is rarely used. The "physiological fundoplication" of Boix Ochoa uses a procedure that increases the angle of His and does an anterior wrap only suturing it to the right crus and then a hitch of the fundus to the left diaphragm. Partial fundoplications are variously described with the wrap only encircling the posterior 180°–270° of the esophagus, and similarly anterior partial fundoplications, encircling part of the anterior part of the esophagus. In those who are neurologically impaired, a partial fundoplication rarely works. They may, however, be appropriate for a second procedure in neurologically intact children, where the first fundoplication produced unrelenting dysphagia that has to be relieved surgically. Even then, they frequently fail. As the child grows, the wraps become looser, so that partial wraps are more likely to fail with time, and tight wraps will slacken, so that dysphagia relents. Laparoscopic fundoplications have largely replaced open approaches. Exceptions occur. The most common would be where there have been multiple abdominal procedures and adhesions; the most extreme would be where neither an open abdominal nor a laparoscopic procedure can be achieved. An example would be after an exomphalos major repair at birth, where the liver now overlies the stomach and is attached to the spleen with adhesions, making access to the upper stomach impossible through the abdomen alone, where a thoracoabdominal approach is often necessary. Dysphagia is frequent early but declines to 5–10 % by 6 months. Similarly, gas bloat syndrome is higher early on but improves over the years. Inability to vomit or belch is much higher in the pediatric population, but is diminishing as the wraps are now shorter and looser. Dysphagia, gas bloat syndrome, and inability to vomit or belch reflect a too tight wrap. Persistent gastroesophageal reflux in pediatrics, which reflects failure or excessive looseness of the wrap, is about 5–10 % for otherwise normal children, but as high as 30–50 % in neurologically impaired children. The incidence of hiatus hernia, including or excluding the wrap, is high in children where (in days gone by) the hiatus was not closed behind the esophagus. There is probably a 15 % increased lifetime risk of hiatus hernia, and this could be as high as 20 % in the first 5 years in those who are neurologically impaired, but again closing the hiatus has reduced this substantially. Breakdown of the fundoplication occurs in about 1–5 % of cases overall, but up to 50 % in neurologically impaired patients. Similarly, delayed gastric emptying occurs in ~1–5 % of cases, but increases to around 20 % of neurologically impaired patients.

**Major Complications**

The most common major complication is **aphagia**, or very severe **dysphagia**, which can occasionally require very **early reoperation** (within days). **Persistent or recurrent gastroesophageal reflux** can occur after failure of the surgery either initially or later, with loosening of the wrap. Damage to the spleen that requires **splenectomy** is very rare in children, and splenic injury occurs far less frequently in laparoscopic surgery than in open surgery. Full-thickness **esophageal or gastric** damage is a major complication, but this occurs very infrequently indeed; in primary antireflux surgery, it is usually seen immediately and repaired immediately. **Infection and multisystem failure** are very rare, but a late perforation or undetected leak can occur to cause this. **Bleeding** is rare and is usually controlled at surgery. **Gas embolus** and **major vascular injury** are additional serious, although very rare, complications of the laparoscopic approach. **Conversion to open operation** is a small but significant risk rather than a complication per se.

---

**Consent and Risk Reduction**

**Main Points to Explain**

- GA risk
- Pain/discomfort
- Bleeding/hematoma*
- Infection (local/systemic)*
- Risk of other abdominal organ injury*
- Intraperitoneal leakage
- Gas embolism
- Conversion to open surgery
- Dysphagia
- Recurrence of reflux
- Possible further surgery*
- Risks without surgery*

  *Dependent on pathology, comorbidities, and surgery performed

---

## Open Appendectomy

### Description

General anesthesia is used. The patient is positioned in the supine position and is best examined when anesthetized to assess whether there is a mass. This may influence the decision to carry out an open (more likely with a mass) procedure or laparoscopic procedure and to determine the best site for the incision, if there is a mass. Rectal examination under anesthesia may be useful to assess the presence of any pelvic mass. Nevertheless, an ultrasound may have been performed. The objective of the operation is to remove the appendix. If, at laparotomy, the appendix does not appear to be inflamed, then the next objective is to determine if there is other pathology by examining the pelvis for pelvic pathology, particularly in the female, and the terminal ileum for the presence of a Meckel's diverticulum or other pathology causing local peritonitis. If there is a large mass, then open appendectomy should be carried out in children, as interval appendectomy does not appear to be warranted. In children, it is rare to be unable to gain access to other pathology from an extended RIF incision. Under most circumstances the appendix can be removed using a small transverse (Lanz) skin incision and a muscle-splitting incision of the internal oblique muscle. A small incision is often made to obtain a good cosmetic result. Surgeons should never hesitate to increase the length of the skin incision and either divide the internal oblique muscle or cut the anterior rectus fascia, retracting the rectus to the midline and opening the posterior rectus sheath after dealing with the inferior epigastric vessels, or both, to provide better access to the peritoneal cavity. Under these circumstances, the cecum should be mobilized by dividing the congenital adhesions to bring the cecum well into the wound to display the full length of the appendix, particularly its junction with the cecum.

## Anatomical Points

The appendix origin lies at the confluence of the taenia coli; however, its tip can vary enormously in position, lying retrocecally (~75 % cases), pelvic (20 %), or retro-ileal/pre-ileal (5 %). The length of the appendix varies also and can reach the upper ascending colon posteriorly. Rarely the appendix (very rare) and cecum may enter a large inguinal hernial sac. Irritation of the bladder or colon can cause urinary urgency and/or diarrhea. An inflamed appendix, if retrocecal or pelvic in location, may irritate the ureter, so that hematuria or dysuria may occur. Irritation of the psoas muscle by an inflamed retrocecal appendix or abscess may cause hip discomfort on movement. Maldescent of the appendix is rare due to malrotation of the cecum, which remains high in the hepatic region. Agenesis, duplication, and situs inversus (left-sided appendix) are exceedingly rare, but can occur. There are, however, a series of patients with left atrial isomerism (picked up on antenatal scans) who are known to have situs inversus.

## Perspective

See Table 3.20. Infective complications are the most common following appendectomy, wound infection being the most frequent. This is often avoided by adequate exposure, preoperative prophylactic antibiotics, and copious lavage of the abdominal cavity and the wound with large volumes of warm saline (usually with an antibiotic in the solution in children). In grossly contaminated (dirty) wounds, the use of drainage of the pelvis and wound, delayed primary skin closure, or the use of gauze pledgets impregnated with antiseptic may be used in an effort to reduce the risk of infection, but this is very rarely needed in children. Abscess formation can occur in the pelvis, right paracolic gutter, between loops of small bowel, or occasionally subphrenic space, usually from preexisting peritonitis. In children, approximately 1/3 of patients will have perforated within 24 h of the onset of symptoms. Damage to anatomical structures in the region rarely occurs in children, but the ilioinguinal or iliohypogastric nerves as they traverse close to the incision or the inferior epigastric vessels may be damaged. Damage to the ovary and right fallopian tube, however, is a well-recognized complication in the young female with peritonitis, either from sepsis or iatrogenically, and infertility may result. Right inguinal hernia and right femoral hernia are more common after appendectomy. Different techniques of dealing with the appendix stump can avoid complications associated

**Table 3.20** Open appendectomy estimated frequency of complications, risks, and consequences

| Complications, risks, and consequences | Estimated frequency |
|---|---|
| *Most significant/serious complications* | |
| Infection[a] | 5–20 % |
| Subcutaneous | 5–20 % |
|   Intra-abdominal/pelvic (peritonitis; abscess) (especially in the very young) | 5–20 % |
|   Systemic sepsis | 2–5 % |
| Especially in the young | |
|   Hepatic portal sepsis (rare) | <0.1 % |
| Bleeding/hematoma formation[a] | |
|   Wound | 1–5 % |
|   Intra-abdominal | 0.1–1 % |
| Small bowel obstruction (early or late)[a] [Adhesion formation] | 1–5 % |
| *Rare significant/serious problems* | |
| Nerve parasthesia | 0.1–1 % |
|   Iliohypogastric/ilioinguinal nerve | |
| Inguinal hernia (right side) | 0.1–1 % |
| Fallopian tube obstruction[a] (right; left very rare) – overall | 0.1–1 % |
|   After pelvic sepsis[b] | 1–5 % |
| Female infertility[a] – overall[c] | <0.1 % |
|   After pelvic sepsis[c, b] | 0.1–1 % |
| Fecal fistula[a] (very rare) | <0.1 % |
| Ureteric injury (very rare)[a] | <0.1 % |
| Multisystem organ failure (renal, pulmonary, cardiac failure) | 0.1–1 % |
| Mortality | <0.1 % |
| Mortality without surgery (should surgery be refused) | >80 % |
| *Less serious complications* | |
| Pain/tenderness | |
|   Acute (<4 weeks) | 5–20 % |
|   Chronic (>4 weeks) | <0.1 % |
| Paralytic ileus (peritonitis from preoperative perforation) | 20–30 % |
| Wound scarring (poor cosmesis/wound deformity)[a] | 1–5 % |
| Nasogastric tube[a] | 1–5 % |
| Wound drain tube(s)[a] | 1–5 % |

[a]Dependent on underlying pathology, anatomy, surgical technique, and preferences
[b]Fallopian tubal obstruction unilaterally may be as high as 8 %; lower bilaterally
[c]The rate of female infertility is related to the extent of perforation, abscess formation, and pelvic sepsis

with the stump including intraperitoneal abscess, "recurrent" appendicitis, and fecal fistula from breakdown of the wound closure of the cecum (stump abscess). Moreover, long-term complications of small bowel obstructions with adhesions, either to the appendix base or to the aperture of the appendix mesentery can occur. Inversion of the stump has been associated with increased risk of small bowel obstruction. Firm suture transfixion/ligation of the appendix base against the cecum usually avoids appendix stump complications.

**Major Complications**

**Abscess formation, fistula or sinus formation**, and **systemic sepsis** are serious complications that may rarely lead to **multisystem organ failure** and even mortality. Early surgery and preoperative antibiotics have reduced these complications significantly. Preexisting comorbidities include established generalized peritonitis and immunosuppression, which can increase risk of infection greatly. **Short-term failure to feed** may indicate **ongoing sepsis. Severe bleeding** is rare and transfusion uncommon. Concealed postoperative bleeding is rare. Persistent **wound sinuses** and a **fecal fistula** are very rare and require prolonged hospitalization and dressings, but most close within 2 months. **Prolonged ileus** and later (even decades later) **small bowel adhesive obstruction** can occur, but are surprisingly uncommon even with extensive adhesions. **Ureteric injury** and **iliac arterial injury** are exceedingly rare, but can be catastrophic. Scarring/adhesions from infection and inflammation can be associated with **fallopian tube obstruction**, tubal non-patency, ectopic or tubal pregnancy, ovarian or tubal torsion, infertility, and adhesional bowel obstruction, depending on the pathology and extent of sepsis.

*Consent and Risk Reduction*

**Main Points to Explain**

- GA risk
- Pain/discomfort
- Bleeding/hematoma*
- Infection (wound/abscess/systemic)*
- Risk of other abdominal organ injury*
- Intraperitoneal leakage
- Possible further surgery*
- Risks without surgery*

  **\*Dependent on pathology, comorbidities, and surgery performed**

# Laparoscopic Appendectomy

### Description

For those with reasonable experience in laparoscopy, appendicitis can be dealt with laparoscopically. General anesthesia is used. The patient is positioned in the supine position and is best examined when anesthetized to assess whether there is a mass to determine whether or not to proceed with the laparoscopy or whether to carry out an open procedure. Initial experience with laparoscopic appendectomy in the presence of an inflammatory mass was associated with a higher incidence of postoperative ileus and intra-abdominal sepsis. That difference in outcome seems to be reducing as experience increases. Rectal examination under anesthesia may be useful to assess the presence of any pelvic mass. The objective of the operation is to remove the appendix. If the appendix is not inflamed, then the pelvis needs examination for pelvic pathology, particularly in the female, and the terminal ileum for the presence of a Meckel's diverticulum or other pathology causing local peritonitis. Occasionally, the inflammatory process, phlegmon, or abscess is so extensive the appendix cannot be removed, and it is judicious to convert to an open procedure. Drainage alone is very rarely used in children. If other pathology is encountered, determining whether to continue laparoscopically, will depend on the pathology. For example, Crohn's disease affecting the terminal ileum and cecum may necessitate open laparotomy.

**Anatomical Points**

The appendix origin lies at the confluence of the taenia coli; however, its tip can vary enormously in position, lying retrocecally (~75 % cases), pelvic (20 %), or retro-ileal/pre-ileal (5 %). The length of the appendix varies also and can reach the upper ascending colon posteriorly. Rarely the appendix (very rare) and cecum may enter a large inguinal hernial sac. Irritation of the bladder or colon can cause urinary urgency and/or diarrhea. An inflamed appendix, if retrocecal or pelvic in location, may irritate the ureter, so that hematuria or dysuria may occur. Irritation of the psoas muscle by an inflamed retrocecal appendix or abscess may cause hip discomfort on movement. Maldescent of the appendix is rare due to malrotation of the cecum, which remains high in the hepatic region. Agenesis, duplication, and situs inversus (left-sided appendix) are exceedingly rare, but can occur. There are, however, a series of patients with left atrial isomerism (picked up on antenatal scans) who are known to have situs inversus.

**Perspective**

See Table 3.21. Infective complications are the most common following appendectomy, wound infection being the most frequent. This is often avoided by adequate exposure, preoperative prophylactic antibiotics, and copious lavage of the abdominal cavity and the wound with large volumes of warm saline (usually with an antibiotic in the solution in children). In grossly contaminated (dirty) wounds, the use of drainage of the pelvis and wound, delayed primary skin closure, or the use of gauze pledgets impregnated with antiseptic may be used in an effort to reduce the risk of infection, but this is very rarely needed in children. Abscess formation can occur in the pelvis, right paracolic gutter, between loops of small bowel, or occasionally subphrenic space, usually from preexisting peritonitis. In children, approximately 1/3 of patients will have perforated within 24 h of the onset of symptoms. Damage to anatomical structures in the region rarely occurs in children, but the ilioinguinal or iliohypogastric nerves as they traverse close to the incision or the

**Table 3.21** Laparoscopic appendectomy estimated frequency of complications, risks, and consequences

| Complications, risks, and consequences | Estimated frequency |
|---|---|
| *Most significant/serious complications* | |
| Infection[a] | 5–20 % |
|   Subcutaneous | 5–20 % |
|   Intra-abdominal/pelvic (peritonitis; abscess) (especially in the very young) | 5–20 % |
|   Systemic sepsis (especially in the young) | 2–5 % |
|   Hepatic portal sepsis (rare) | <0.1 % |
| Bleeding/hematoma formation[a] | |
|   Wound | 1–5 % |
|   Intra-abdominal | 0.1–1 % |
| Small bowel obstruction (early or late)[a] [Adhesion formation] | 1–5 % |
| Conversion to open operation[a] | 1–5 % |
| Extension of wound for access/safety (for improving exposure)[a] | 1–5 % |
| Mortality | <0.1 % |
| Mortality without surgery (should surgery be refused) | >80 % |
| *Rare significant/serious problems* | |
| Nerve parasthesia | 0.1–1 % |
|   Iliohypogastric/ilioinguinal nerve | |
| Gas embolism[a] | <0.1 % |
| Ureteric injury[a] | <0.1 % |
| Vascular injury[a] | <0.1 % |
| Fecal fistula[a] | <0.1 % |
| Inguinal hernia (right side) | 0.1–1 % |
| Multisystem failure (renal, pulmonary, cardiac failure) | 0.1–1 % |
| *Less serious complications* | |
| Pain/tenderness | |
|   Acute (<4 weeks) | 1–5 % |
|   Chronic (>4 weeks) | <0.1 % |
| Paralytic ileus (peritonitis from preoperative perforation) | 20–30 % |
| Wound scarring (poor cosmesis/wound deformity)[a] | 1–5 % |
| Nasogastric tube[a] | 1–5 % |
| Wound drain tube(s)[a] | 1–5 % |

[a]Dependent on underlying pathology, anatomy, surgical technique, and preferences

inferior epigastric vessels may be damaged. Damage to the ovary and right fallopian tube, however, is a well-recognized complication in the young female with peritonitis. Right inguinal hernia and right femoral hernia are more common after appendectomy. Different techniques of dealing with the appendix stump can avoid complications associated with the stump including intraperitoneal abscess, "recurrent" appendicitis, and fecal fistula from breakdown of the wound closure of the cecum (stump abscess). Moreover, long-term complications of small bowel obstructions with adhesions, either to the appendix base or to the aperture of the appendix mesentery can occur. Inversion of the stump has been associated with increased risk of small bowel obstruction. Firm (double) loop ligation of the appendix base against the cecum usually avoids appendix stump complications. Conversion to open laparotomy may be required for a complicated appendix or other pathology. Complications of laparoscopy are relatively very rare, but include gas embolism, vascular or bowel trauma, surgical emphysema, and pneumothorax. Gas embolism is associated with Veress needle insertion, which can virtually be eliminated by open cutdown methods. Pneumothorax is a rare, idiosyncratic complication, probably from diaphragmatic leakage of gas.

## Major Complications

**Abscess formation, fistula or sinus formation**, and **systemic sepsis** are serious complications that may rarely lead to **multisystem organ failure** and even mortality. Early surgery and preoperative antibiotics have reduced these complications significantly. Preexisting comorbidities include established generalized peritonitis and immunosuppression, which can increase the risk of infection greatly. **Short-term failure to feed** may indicate **ongoing sepsis. Severe bleeding** is rare and transfusion uncommon. Concealed postoperative bleeding is rare. Persistent **wound sinuses** and a **fecal fistula** are very rare and require prolonged hospitalization and dressings, but most close within 2 months. **Prolonged ileus** and later (even decades later) **small bowel adhesive obstruction** can occur, but are surprisingly uncommon even with extensive adhesions. **Gas embolism** is a very rare but catastrophic complication. **Ureteric injury** and **iliac arterial injury** are exceedingly rare but can be catastrophic. **Conversion to open operation** is a small but significant risk rather than a complication per se.

**Consent and Risk Reduction**

**Main Points to Explain**

- GA risk
- Pain/discomfort
- Bleeding/hematoma*
- Infection (wound/abscess/systemic)*
- Risk of other abdominal organ injury*
- Intraperitoneal leakage
- Gas embolism
- Conversion to open surgery
- Possible further surgery*
- Risks without surgery*

**\*Dependent on pathology, comorbidities, and surgery performed**

## Surgery for Liver Tumors and Limited Liver Resection (Segmentectomy, Sectorectomy, and Sector Resection)

### Description

General anesthesia is used. The aim of performing a segmental resection is typically to remove a solitary benign or malignant liver tumor, although several lesions may be amenable to segmental resection. Hepatoblastoma (45 %) and hepatocellular carcinoma (25 %) account for most primary malignant liver tumors. Hemangioendothelioma is the most common benign tumor. Although metastatic liver tumors are relatively rare in children, they do occur with Wilms' tumors of the kidney. They can be amenable to resection.

For any resection of a liver tumor, the goal is to achieve clear margins around the lesion(s), as well as excising any liver parenchyma, devascularized from occlusion of segmental portal inflow. Segmental resections can be combined with a contralateral major hepatectomy for complete resection of bilateral disease. Hemihepatectomy or lobectomy may be more appropriate than segmentectomy for livers in small children.

### Anatomical Points

The anatomical variance in the performance of segmentectomy or sectorectomy is primarily dictated by the possible variant inflow that can occur with the right lobe of the liver. The right hepatic inflow that supplies segments 5, 6, 7, and 8 arises from the junction of the right and left portal vein. In a majority of cases, there is a common right portal vein that branches into the right anterior sectorial and right posterior sectorial branches. However, the main right portal vein leading to the right anterior and right posterior sectorial branches may be absent, instead originating at the same junction as the left portal vein. Another main portal anatomic variance can occur with the early take off of the right posterior sectorial vein, with the bifurcation then occurring at the left portal vein and the right anterior sectorial vein. Inflow within the right hepatic lobe can also vary with segment-6 inflow branches originating from the anterior sectorial branches and creating an isolated segment-7 branch. This anatomical variant is important to ensure that only a single segment of inflow is occluded instead of the entire right lobe or the anterior or posterior segment, respectively.

### Perspective

See Table 3.22. Potential major complications of hepatic resection in children are **bleeding, hepatic failure from devascularized liver, and biliary leakage**. **Bleeding** during segmentectomy and sectorectomy primarily occurs from the outflow hepatic veins. These are thin-walled veins that tear easily and can develop

**Table 3.22**  Surgery for liver tumors estimated frequency of complications, risks, and consequences

| Complications, risks, and consequences | Estimated frequency |
|---|---|
| *Most significant/serious complications* | |
| Infection | |
| Wound | 1–5 % |
| Intra-abdominal(including liver/liver bed/subphrenic abscess) | 1–5 % |
| Intrathoracic (pneumonia; pleural) | 5–20 % |
| Mediastinitis (if vena cava isolation used) | 0.1–1 % |
| Systemic | 1–5 % |
| Bleeding/hematoma formation overall | 5–20 % |
| Arterial, venous (caval, renal, portal, hepatic, or lobar vessels) | 1–5 % |
| Raw liver surface | 1–5 % |
| Extrahepatic | 1–5 % |
| Subcapsular hematoma[a] (major) | 1–5 % |
| Serous ascitic collection | 1–5 % |
| Bile duct ischemia | 1–5 % |
| Bile duct stenosis | 1–5 % |
| Biliary obstruction | 5–20 % |
| Bile leak/collection | 5–20 % |
| Biliary ascites | 1–5 % |
| Biliary fistula | 1–5 % |
| Hyperbilirubinemia | 50–80 % |
| Jaundice | 1–5 % |
| Common/extrahepatic/intrahepatic bile duct injury | 1–5 % |
| Unresectability of malignancy or tumor/involved resection margins[a] | Individual |
| Recurrence of malignancy[a] | Individual |
| Bowel injury (stomach, duodenum, small bowel, colon) | 1–5 % |
| Thrombosis | |
| Arterial (hepatic) | 1–5 % |
| Venous (hepatic) | 1–5 % |
| Liver failure (ischemia; toxicity; acute hepatic necrosis) early or late | 5–20 % |
| Liver injury (to remaining liver) | 1–5 % |
| Surgical emphysema[a] (major) | 1–5 % |
| Gastrointestinal erosion, ulceration, perforation, hemorrhage | 1–5 % |
| Small bowel obstruction (early or late)[a] [Ischemic stenosis/adhesion formation] | 1–5 % |
| Reflux esophagitis/pharyngitis/pneumonitis | 1–5 % |
| Coagulopathy | 1–5 % |
| Disseminated intravascular coagulopathy | |
| [a]Consumption transfusion (large bleed) | |
| Pericardial effusion | 1–5 % |
| Muscle weakness (atrophy due to denervation esp subcostal incision) | 1–5 % |
| Nutritional deficiency – anemia, B12 malabsorption[a] | 5–20 % |
| Multisystem failure (renal, pulmonary, cardiac failure) | 1–5 % |
| Mortality[a] | 1–5 % |
| Mortality <u>without</u> surgery[a] (for hepatoblastoma virtually 100 %) | >80 % |

(continued)

**Table 3.22** (continued)

| Complications, risks, and consequences | Estimated frequency |
|---|---|
| *Rare significant/serious problems* | |
| Aspiration pneumonitis | 0.1–1 % |
| Portal venous thrombosis[a] | 0.1–1 % |
| Deep venous thrombosis | 0.1–1 % |
| Air embolus (major) | 0.1–1 % |
| Renal/adrenal injury renal vein | 0.1–1 % |
| Diaphragmatic injury paresis | 0.1–1 % |
| Diaphragmatic hernia | 0.1–1 % |
| Pancreatic injury/pancreatitis/pancreatic cyst/pancreatic fistula | 0.1–1 % |
| Thoracic duct injury (chylous leak, fistula)[a] | 0.1–1 % |
| Budd-Chiari (acute) | 0.1–1 % |
| Splenic injury (conservation (consequent limitation to activity; late rupture) or splenectomy) | 0.1–1 % |
| Hepatitis (drug, CMV, recurrent)[a] | 0.1–1 % |
| Renal failure (hepatorenal syndrome)[a] | 0.1–1 % |
| Hyperglycemia | 0.1–1 % |
| Hypoglycemia | 0.1–1 % |
| Wound dehiscence | 0.1–1 % |
| *Less serious complications* | |
| Pain/tenderness | |
|    Acute (<4 weeks) | 5–20 % |
|    Chronic (>4 weeks) | <0.1 % |
| Incisional hernia formation (delayed heavy lifting) | 1–5 % |
| Paralytic ileus | 20–50 % |
| Nasogastric tube[a] | 1–5 % |
| Blood transfusion[a] | 5–20 % |
| Wound drain tube(s)[a] | Individual |
| Wound scarring (poor cosmesis/wound deformity) | 1–5 % |

[a]Dependent on underlying pathology, anatomy, surgical technique, and preferences

lateral tears, which can extend up to the main venous branches or to the inferior vena cava underneath intact hepatic parenchyma. Thus, any form of segmentectomy or sectorial resection must identify all of the major hepatic venous outflow structures to ensure adequate hemostasis and to minimize blood loss. **Biliary leakage** is primarily a problem in patients who are undergoing some form of bile duct resection and require biliary reconstruction. Biliary leakage is less common when performing a segmentectomy or sectorectomy and primarily will occur because of the inadvertent transection of a (small) bile duct without adequate closure. The performance of a segmentectomy should not be automatically assumed to be a lesser operative procedure compared to hepatic lobectomy or some form of extended hepatic lobectomy. There have been recent evaluations showing that intraoperative blood loss is significantly greater when a segmentectomy is performed, compared to an anatomic hepatic lobectomy. The reason for this is principally difficulty with small venous outflow control that may lead to increased blood loss during the resection phase. All segmental resections are not of similar difficulty. A segment-3 resection is technically far easier, compared to a segment-8 resection. The anatomical variation, the depth of the liver parenchyma, and the patient body habitus can make various types of segmental resections more difficult in certain patients.

## Major Complications

**Intraoperative bleeding** during a segmentectomy can be the most serious complication because of injury without ligation of the outflow hepatic veins. If the central venous pressure (CVP) is not low, the risk of intraoperative hemorrhage is increased. Hepatic venous outflow hemorrhage from inadvertent transection of the hepatic veins primarily occurs because of the inability to identify anatomic variations intraoperatively. **Intraoperative air embolus** can be a severe and life-threatening complication due to inadvertent laceration of the hepatic veins during hepatic parenchymal transection, with aspiration of air into the vena cava. This complication can be related to low CVP while parenchymal transection is performed. Hence, optimal controlled hypotension with a CVP of 0–1 cm $H_2O$ has been proven to be the most effective anesthetic management in patients who undergo any form of hepatic resection. The acute management of a patient who has sustained an air embolus is immediate steep Trendelenburg (head-down) position, with occlusion of the parenchymal transection site with a wet laparotomy gauze pack and aggressive support measures by the anesthetist. This complication can be effectively prevented by ensuring identification and proper ligation of all hepatic venous branches prior to transection. **Postoperative bile leakage** after a segmentectomy or sectorectomy can also lead to significant morbidity, depending on the extent of injury. A recent prospective randomized controlled trial has shown that intraoperative drains placed in patients undergoing hepatic resections do not lead to decreased perioperative morbidity or lessen the need for subsequent postoperative drainage. Thus, meticulous intraoperative hemostasis, as well as identification and ligation of all bile ducts during hepatic transection cannot be overemphasized. Omentoplasty has been utilized to prevent bile leakage after resection; however, in a recent prospective randomized controlled trial, this technique was not found to significantly reduce bile leakage. Further review of this report also showed that omentoplasty did not adversely affect the patient either; thus, the utilization should be surgeon determined. The vast majority of patients who sustain a postoperative bile leak either resolve spontaneously or can be managed with a percutaneous drainage and bedside supportive care.

**Devascularization:** In the small child with a hepatoblastoma, the vessels are small so that small segmental arteries may go into vasospasm, or they can be inadvertently injured in the porta hepatis, even using bipolar diathermy. This can even be seen to the residual arterial supply after major hepatic resection, and especially so with the Kasai procedure, when the patient is only weeks old, where extensive dissection in the porta hepatis is paramount to get an extended resection of the hepatic plate. So, all of the arterial supply is at risk.

**Tumor recurrence** following resection of a hepatic malignancy is a significant problem and is integrally related to the width of resection margin of normal liver around the lesions(s). Tumor rupture may occur preoperatively or intraoperatively especially with large, necrotic tumors. Tumor leakage may disseminate tumor and worsen the prognosis. Development of further tumor metastases after metastasectomy arising from previously subclinical micrometastases is another limitation to successful surgical treatment. Although these are not strictly complications per se, they are contingent on effective preoperative evaluation and surgical technique. **Infection** of the wound or peritoneal cavity (**peritonitis, abscess**) can lead to sepsis and **multisystem organ failure** and significant **mortality**. Respiratory and cardiac complications are moderately common and are increased if anomalies are present. **Liver failure** can result from a long operative ischemic time. **Recurrence of tumor** depends heavily on the pathology and further metastasis. If a hepatoblastoma is not fully resected, then death is almost inevitable despite aggressive chemotherapy. In those circumstances, if the tumor is thought to be unresectable, it may be better to plan a liver transplant, as metastases do not appear to occur early when the child is having chemotherapy. At the initial presentation, hepatoblastomas often look unresectable, but with chemotherapy, they may become resectable with conventional techniques.

---

**Consent and Risk Reduction**

**Main Points to Explain**

- GA risk
- Pain/discomfort
- Bleeding/hematoma*
- Infection (local/systemic)*
- Risk of other abdominal organ injury*
- Intraperitoneal leakage
- Air embolism
- Possible further surgery*
- Recurrence of tumor
- Risks without surgery*
- Multisystem organ failure
- Death

  ***Dependent on pathology, comorbidities, and surgery performed**

---

# Open Splenectomy

## Description

General anesthesia is used. The aim is to electively remove the spleen, including any small remnant splenunculi, which may be separate from the main splenic mass.

The degree of difficulty and relative risk of complications is proportional to the size of the spleen and underlying disease process. A midline, left subcostal, or left transverse upper abdominal incision is usual. The spleen is mobilized on its pedicle, freeing any adhesions with the abdominal wall or organs. The short gastric vessels often require division specifically. Occasionally, the splenic flexure of the colon overlies the spleen and needs to be "taken down" to permit better exposure. In general, the spleen is freed from attachments to surrounding structures and is then lifted and rotated anteromedially toward the right side to expose the splenic hilum from behind. A clamp(s) is then placed across the splenic pedicle, divided then ligated, taking care not to injure the pancreatic tail. Individual vessels can be identified easily in children, so each artery can be ligated, followed by the veins. The spleen can then be delivered through the abdominal incision and removed. The pedicle and splenic bed are checked and hemostasis is achieved. A drain may be used, more for possible pancreatic leakage than bleeding. Accessory splenic tissue is sought (splenunculi), particularly in patients with idiopathic thrombocytopenic purpura (ITP), and removed as each can grow to a degree that allows disease recurrence. Removal of the spleen for severe trauma or surgical rupture carries a different spectrum of risk, should conservative management not be possible or appropriate. In children a standard layered closure with absorbable sutures is usually used.

**Anatomical Points**

The spleen may be lobulated as a normal variant, as embryologically, it forms from fusion of individual lobules. A fissure may even occur with two or more separate lobes or separate spleens. Small, usually rounded, deposits of splenic tissue may exist as splenunculi, often around the splenic hilum, vessels within the lesser sac, or omentum. The short gastric vessels may be closely applied to the spleen, making division difficult and the risk of injury greater especially at the upper pole. Adhesions to the anterior, lateral, or posterior abdominal wall, diaphragm, or bowel may occur. The splenic flexure of the colon may be tethered to the spleen or above to the lateral abdominal wall, reducing access. The tail of pancreas may overlie the splenic hilum where it is at risk of injury and may also impede access. The splenic vessels may be multiple and widely separated, requiring several individual ligations. The kidney is usually easily separated from the spleen, but can be adherent on occasions, particularly with malignant involvement or severe inflammatory processes. An enlarged spleen can migrate toward the right iliac fossa and render access to the hilum and delivery difficult.

**Perspective**

See Table 3.23. Splenectomy can be an elective procedure (eg. small spleen in ITP, or a moderate-sized to massive spleen for hematological disorders or metastatic malignancy) or an acute procedure (eg. hemorrhage from splenic trauma in a shocked patient). Note that conservative management of splenic trauma is the norm for children, and laparotomy is rarely used for isolated splenic trauma.

**Table 3.23** Open splenectomy estimated frequency of complications, risks, and consequences

| Complications, risks, and consequences | Estimated frequency |
|---|---|
| *Most significant/serious complications* | |
| Infection[a] | |
|   Subcutaneous | 1–5 % |
|   Wound | 1–5 % |
|   Intra-abdominal | 0.1–1 % |
|   Chest infection | 1–5 % |
|   Subphrenic abscess[a] | 0.1–1 % |
|   Late – overwhelming post-splenectomy sepsis (with vaccination) lifetime risk | 5–10 % |
|   Mortality from post-splenectomy sepsis | 1–5 % |
| Bleeding/hematoma formation[b] | 0.1–1 % |
| Small bowel obstruction (early or late)[a] | 1–5 % |
| Excessive NG losses (usually lasting no more than 5 days) | 5–20 % |
| *Rare significant/serious problems* | |
| Pancreatic injury/pancreatitis/pancreatic cyst/leakage/pancreatic fistula | 0.1–1 % |
| Bowel injury (stomach, duodenum, small bowel, colon)[b] | 0.1–1 % |
| Renal/adrenal injury[a] | 0.1–1 % |
| Diaphragmatic injury[a] | 0.1–1 % |
| Accessory spleen formation[b] (Mainly ITP; trauma) | 0.1–1 % |
| Mortality without surgery[c] | Variable |
| *Less serious complications* | |
| Pain/tenderness | |
|   Acute (<4 weeks) | 5–20 % |
|   Chronic (>4 weeks) | <0.1 % |
| Paralytic ileus[b] | 5–20 % |
| Incisional hernia (avoid lifting/straining for 8/52) | 0.1–1 % |
| Wound scarring (deformity/dimpling of wound scar/poor cosmesis) | 1–5 % |
| Drain tube(s)[a] | 5–20 % |

[a]Dependent on underlying pathology, surgical technique preferences, and location on the body
[b]Incidence may be higher for moderate and massive splenomegaly
[c]Depending on the underlying disease; much higher for malignancy. NB: The spectrum of risk following trauma is different

The degree of difficulty can vary markedly between these situations as can the risks and complications. Spill of splenic tissue (e.g., with rupture) can lead to recurrent ITP or malignancy, depending on the initial pathology and situation. Infection is more common in malignant conditions, in immunocompromised individuals, and after multi-trauma, especially if preexisting or concurrent lung trauma or infection is present. Infection of a hematoma in the splenic bed may result in a subphrenic abscess. Inadvertent injury to the bowel or pancreas may result in infection or a fistula, which can be chronic and debilitating, with slow closure. Overwhelming post-splenectomy pneumonia or sepsis carries a lifetime risk of up to 2–10 % of those that have a hematological reason for the splenectomy and 1 % of those after trauma. Vaccination does not give adequate protection for all strains of pathogens, especially pneumococcus, but may be effective for hemophilus, so that "overwhelming post-splenectomy infection (OPSI)" still occurs. So, parent/patient must be educated to seek medical advice immediately the baby/child/adult appears to be mildly infected. Often, an early megadose of penicillin is very effective. Paralytic ileus is common but usually resolves spontaneously within a week. Injury to the adrenal and kidney is very rare. Excessive nasogastric loses frequently occur for several days after surgery, possibly as a result of division of the short gastric vessels.

## Major Complications

**Respiratory infection** is perhaps the most common complication and may lead to lobar **pneumonia** and **severe systemic sepsis**. **Bleeding** and ongoing **oozing** can be significant, especially in patients with coagulopathies; however, hemostasis at surgery usually controls this adequately. **Recurrent ITP** can be a problem, if ITP was the reason for splenectomy, and may require intraoperative nuclear scans and further surgery. **Recurrent malignancy** can also occur, if tumor or blood spill occurs during splenectomy for malignancy. The use of a plastic bag around the spleen before splenic ligation may reduce the risk of both forms of recurrence. **Wound infection, peritonitis,** and **intra-abdominal abscess formation** may predispose to **wound dehiscence** and even "burst" abdomen. **Pancreatic leakage, pseudocyst formation,** and **fistula formation** are relatively uncommon, but can be very debilitating. **Small bowel obstruction** is not uncommon even years after surgery. **Overwhelming post-splenectomy sepsis** is a rare, potentially serious later complication.

---

**Consent and Risk Reduction**

**Main Points to Explain**

- GA risk
- Bleeding/hematoma
- Infection (local/systemic)
- Pain/discomfort
- Possible tumor recurrence*
- Other abdominal organ injury
- Respiratory complications
- Venous thromboembolism
- Possible blood transfusion
- Risks without surgery

   **\*Dependent on pathology and type of surgery performed**

# Laparoscopic Splenectomy

## Description

General anesthesia is used. The aim is to remove the spleen, using laparoscopic techniques, including any small remnant splenunculi, which may be separate from the main splenic mass. The degree of difficulty and relative risk of complications is proportional to the size of the spleen and underlying disease process. A range of patient positions have been used, including the right lateral decubitus, but the usual to have the left sided elevated to 30°–45°. Ports are then placed and the procedure performed. A small midline, left subcostal, or left transverse upper abdominal incision may be used in conjunction for larger or difficult spleens. The spleen is mobilized on its pedicle, freeing any adhesions with the abdominal wall or organs. The short gastric vessels will often require division specifically. Occasionally, the splenic flexure of the colon overlies the spleen and needs to be "taken down" to permit better exposure. In general, the spleen is freed from attachments to surrounding structures and is then lifted laterally to the left side to expose the splenic hilum from in front. A vascular stapling device(s) is then placed across the splenic pedicle, which ligated and divided, taking care not to injure the pancreatic tail. The spleen can then be placed in a plastic bag, delivered through an abdominal incision, or morcellated (minced) and removed. The pedicle and splenic bed are checked and hemostasis is achieved. A drain may be used, more for possible pancreatic leakage than bleeding. Accessory splenic tissue is sought, particularly in idiopathic thrombocytopenic purpura (ITP) cases, and removed. Port-site and abdominal closure is usually performed.

## Anatomical Points

The spleen may be lobulated as a normal variant, as embryologically, it forms from fusion of individual lobules. A fissure may even occur with two or more separate lobes, or separate spleens. Small, usually rounded, deposits of splenic tissue may exist as splenunculi, often around the splenic hilum, vessels within the lesser sac, or omentum. The short gastric vessels may be closely applied to the spleen, making division difficult and the risk of injury greater. Adhesions to the anterior, lateral, or posterior abdominal wall, diaphragm, or bowel may occur. The splenic flexure of the colon may be tethered to the spleen or above to the lateral abdominal wall, reducing access. The tail of pancreas may overlie the splenic hilum where it is at risk of injury and may also impede access. The splenic vessels may be multiple and widely separated, requiring several individual ligations. The kidney is usually easily separated from the spleen, but can be adherent on occasions, particularly with malignant involvement or severe inflammatory processes. An enlarged spleen can migrate toward the right iliac fossa and render access to the hilum and delivery difficult.

**Table 3.24** Laparoscopic splenectomy estimated frequency of complications, risks, and consequences

| Complications, risks, and consequences | Estimated frequency |
|---|---|
| ***Most significant/serious complications*** | |
| Infection | |
| Subcutaneous | 1–5 % |
| Wound | 1–5 % |
| Intra-abdominal | 0.1–1 % |
| Late – post-splenectomy sepsis (with vaccination) | 0.1–1 % |
| Chest infection | 1–5 % |
| Subphrenic abscess[a] | 0.1–1 % |
| Late – overwhelming post-splenectomy sepsis (with vaccination) lifetime risk | 5–10 % |
| Mortality from post-splenectomy sepsis | 1–5 % |
| Bleeding/hematoma formation[b] | 0.1–1 % |
| Small bowel obstruction (early or late)[a] | 1–5 % |
| Excessive NG losses (usually lasting no more than 5 days) | 5–20 % |
| Conversion to open surgical procedure[b] | 1–5 % |
| ***Rare significant/serious problems*** | |
| Gas embolus | 0.1–1 % |
| Pancreatic injury/pancreatitis/pancreatic cyst/leakage/pancreatic fistula | 0.1–1 % |
| Bowel injury (stomach, duodenum, small bowel, colon) | 0.1–1 % |
| Renal/adrenal injury | 0.1–1 % |
| Diaphragmatic injury | 0.1–1 % |
| Small bowel obstruction (early or late) | 0.1–1 % |
| Subphrenic abscess | 0.1–1 % |
| Accessory spleen formation[b] | 0.1–1 % |
| (mainly ITP trauma) | |
| Mortality without surgery[c] | Variable |
| ***Less serious complications*** | |
| Pain/tenderness | |
| Acute (<4 weeks) | 5–20 % |
| Chronic (>4 weeks) | <0.1 % |
| Paralytic ileus[b] | 5–20 % |
| Port-site hernia (s) (avoid lifting/straining) | 0.1–1 % |
| Wound scarring (deformity/dimpling of wound scar/poor cosmesis) | 1–5 % |
| Drain tube(s)[a] | 5–20 % |

[a]Dependent on underlying pathology, surgical technique preferences, and location on the body
[b]Incidence may be higher for moderate and massive splenomegaly
[c]Depending on the underlying disease; much higher for malignancy

## Perspective

See Table 3.24. Splenectomy can range from an elective procedure with a small spleen in ITP, for a moderate-sized spleen, or massive spleen for hematological disorders or metastatic malignancy to an acute procedure for hemorrhage from splenic trauma in a shocked patient. But, open surgery is more likely to be used for massive splenic trauma, where there may be liver damage as well. Note that conservative management of splenic trauma is the norm for children, and laparotomy is rarely used for isolated splenic trauma. The degree of difficulty can vary markedly between these situations as can the risks and complications. Spill of splenic tissue (e.g., with rupture) can lead to recurrent ITP or malignancy, depending on the initial pathology and situation. Infection is more common in malignant conditions, in immunocompromised individuals, and after multi-trauma, especially if preexisting or concurrent lung trauma or infection is present. Infection of a hematoma in the splenic bed may result in a subphrenic abscess. Inadvertent injury to the bowel or pancreas may result in infection or a fistula, which can be chronic and debilitating, with slow closure. Overwhelming post-splenectomy pneumonia or sepsis carries a lifetime risk of up to 2 % of those that have a hematological reason for the splenectomy and 1 % of those after trauma. Vaccination does not give adequate protection for all strains of pathogens, especially pneumococcus, but may be effective for hemophilus, so that "overwhelming post-splenectomy infection (OPSI)" still occurs. So, parent/patient must be educated to seek medical advice immediately the baby/child/adult appears to be mildly infected. Often, an early megadose of penicillin is very effective. Paralytic ileus is common but usually resolves spontaneously within a week. Injury to the adrenal and kidney is very rare. Excessive nasogastric loses frequently occur for several days after surgery, possibly as a result of division of the short gastric vessels.

## Major Complications

**Respiratory infection** is perhaps the most common complication and may lead to lobar **pneumonia** and **severe systemic sepsis**. **Bleeding** and ongoing **oozing** can be significant, especially in patients with coagulopathies; however, hemostasis at surgery usually controls this adequately. **Recurrent ITP** can be a problem, if ITP was the reason for splenectomy, and may require intraoperative nuclear scans and further surgery. **Recurrent malignancy** can also occur, if tumor or blood spill occurs during splenectomy for malignancy. The use of a plastic bag around the spleen before splenic ligation may reduce the risk of both forms of recurrence. **Wound infection, peritonitis,** and **intra-abdominal abscess formation** may predispose to **wound dehiscence** and even "burst" abdomen. **Pancreatic leakage, pseudocyst formation,** and **fistula formation** are relatively uncommon, but can be very debilitating. **Small bowel obstruction** is not uncommon even years after surgery. **Overwhelming post-splenectomy sepsis** is a rare, potentially serious later complication. Laparoscopic **injury to bowel or blood vessels** is uncommon, although greater than for open splenectomy, and **gas embolism** although potentially catastrophic is very rare.

**Consent and Risk Reduction**

**Main Points to Explain**

- GA risk
- Bleeding/hematoma
- Infection (local/systemic)
- Pain/discomfort
- Possible tumor recurrence*
- Other abdominal organ injury
- Respiratory complications
- Venous thromboembolism
- Possible blood transfusion
- Gas embolism
- Possible open operation
- Risks without surgery

**\*Dependent on pathology and type of surgery performed**

# Further Reading, References, and Resources

# General Reading[1] [2]

Ellis H. Clinical anatomy. 11th ed. Blackwell; Oxford, 2006.

Jamieson GG, editor. The anatomy of general surgical operations. Edinburgh: Churchill-Livingstone Elsevier; 2006. ISBN 9780443100079.

Moore KL. The developing human: clinically oriented embryology. 2nd ed. Philadelphia: WB Saunders; 1977. ISBN 0-7216-6471-7.

Scott-Conner CEH, Dawson DL. Operative anatomy. 3rd ed. Philadelphia: Lippincott Williams & Wilkins; 2008. ISBN 97807817653.

Skandalakis LJ, Skandalakis JE, Skandalakis 3rd PN, editors. Surgical anatomy and technique: a pocket manual. 3rd ed. New York: Springer; 2009. ISBN 9780387095141.

Ashcraft KW, Holcomb GW, Murphy JP, editors. Ashcraft's pediatric surgery. 5th ed. Philadelphia: Saunders/Elsevier; 2009. ISBN 9781416061274.

Caty MG. Complications in pediatric surgery. New York: Informa Healthcare; 2008. ISBN 9780824728366.

Grant HW, Chuturgoon AA, Kenoyer DG, Doorasamy T. The adaptive immune response to major surgery in the neonate. Pediatr Surg Int. 1997;12(7):490–3.

---

[1] Embryology and Operative Anatomy

[2] Operative Surgery

Grosfeld JL, editor. Pediatric surgery. 6th ed. Philadelphia: Elsevier Science; 2006. ISBN 9780323028424.

Harmon CM, Coran AG. Congenital anomalies of the esophagus, associated anomalies, Ch 62. In: O'Neill Jr JA, Rowe MI, Grosfeld JL, Fonkalsrud EW, Coran AG, editors. Pediatric surgery. 5th ed. St Louis: Mosby Press; 1998. p. 945–6.

Hutson JM, O'Brien M, Woodward AA, Beasley SW. Clinical paediatric surgery: diagnosis & management. 6th ed. Melbourne: Wiley-Blackwell; 2008. ISBN 978-1405162678.

O'Neill Jr JA, Rowe MI, Grosfeld JL, Fonkalsrud EW, Coran AG, editors. Pediatric surgery. 5th ed. St Louis: Mosby Press; 1998.

Spitz L, Coran AG, editors. Operative pediatric surgery. 6th ed. London: Hodder-Arnold; 2006.

Puri P, editor. Newborn surgery. 2nd ed. London: Arnold; 2003. ISBN 9780340761441.

Rowe MI. The newborn as a surgical patient, Ch 4. In: O'Neill Jr JA, Rowe MI, Grosfeld JL, Fonkalsrud EW, Coran AG, editors. Pediatric surgery. 5th ed. St Louis: Mosby Press; 1998. p. 43–70.

Stringer MD, Oldham KT, Moriguard PDE. Pediatric surgery and urology. 2nd ed. Cambridge: Cambridge University Press; 2006a. ISBN 9780521839020.

Stringer MD, Oldham KT, Mouriquand PDE. Pediatric surgery and urology: long-term outcomes. Cambridge: Cambridge University Press; 2006b.

Welch KJ, Randolph JG, Ravitch MM, et al., editors. Pediatric surgery. 5th ed. Chicago: Year Book Medical; 1998.

# More Specific Reading [3][4][5][6][7][8][9][10]

van Eijck FC, Wijnen RM, van Goor HJ. The incidence and morbidity of adhesions after treatment of neonates with gastroschisis and omphalocele: a 30-year review. Pediatr Surg. 2008;43(3):479–83.

Albanese CT, Rowe MI. Necrotizing enterocolitis, Ch 87. In: O'Neill Jr JA, Rowe MI, Grosfeld JL, Fonkalsrud EW, Coran AG, editors. Pediatric surgery. 5th ed. St Louis: Mosby Press; 1998. p. 1297–320.

Boix-Ochoa J, Rowe MI. Gastroesophageal reflux, Ch 66. In: O'Neill Jr JA, Rowe MI, Grosfeld JL, Fonkalsrud EW, Coran AG, editors. Pediatric surgery. 5th ed. St Louis: Mosby Press; 1998. p. 1007–17.

Chacko J, Ford WDA, Haslam R. Neurological developmental outcome in very low birth weight infants after laparotomy. Pediatr Surg Int. 1999;15:496–9.

Cole C, Freitas A, Clifton MS, Durham MM. Hereditary multiple intestinal atresias: 2 new cases and review of the literature. J Pediatr Surg. 2010;45(4):E21–4.

Dalla Vecchia LK, Grosfeld JL, West KW, Rescorla FJ, Scherer LR, Engum SA. Intestinal atresia and stenosis: a 25-year experience with 277 cases. Arch Surg. 1998;133(5):490–6; discussion 496–7. Review.

---

[3] Gastroschisis and Omphalocele

[4] Atresia and Gut Obstructions

[5] Congenital Diaphragmatic Hernia

[6] Hirschsprung's and Anorectal Malformations

[7] Fundoplications

[8] Hernia Repair

[9] Gastrotomy

[10] Splenectomy

Efrati O, Nir J, Fraser D, Cohen-Cymberknoh M, Shoseyov D, Vilozni D, Modan-Moses D, Levy R, Szeinberg A, Kerem E, Rivlin J. Meconium ileus in patients with cystic fibrosis is not a risk factor for clinical deterioration and survival: the Israeli multicenter study. J Pediatr Gastroenterol Nutr. 2010;50(2):173–8.

Federici S, Domenichelli V, Antonellini C, Dòmini R. Multiple intestinal atresia with apple peel syndrome: successful treatment by five end-to-end anastomoses, jejunostomy, and transanastomotic silicone stent. J Pediatr Surg. 2003;38(8):1250–2.

Khong TY, Ford WDA, Haan EA. Umbilical cord ulceration in association with intestinal atresia in a child with deletion 13q and Hirschsprung's disease. Arch Dis Child. 1994;71:F212–3.

Messina M, Molinaro F, Ferrara F, Messina G, Di Maggio G. Idiopathic spontaneous intestinal perforation: a distinct pathological entity in the preterm infant. Minerva Pediatr. 2009;61(4): 355–60.

Murphy FL, Sparnon AL. Long-term complications following intestinal malrotation and the Ladd's procedure: a 15 year review. Pediatr Surg Int. 2006;22(4):326–9.

Ooi BC, Barnes GL, Tauro GP. Normalization of vitamin B12 absorption after ileal resection in children. J Paediatr Child Health. 1992;28(2):168–71.

Pueyo C, Maldonado J, Royo Y, Skrabski R, Di Crosta I, Raventós A. Intrauterine intussusception: a rare cause of intestinal atresia. J Pediatr Surg. 2009;44(10):2028–30.

Rausin L, Khamis J, Paquot JP, Langhendries JP. Obstruction of unusual origin in a small preterm baby-girl. J Belge Radiol. 1992;75(5):402–3.

Rescorla FJ. Meconium ileus, Ch 75. In: O'Neill Jr JA, Rowe MI, Grosfeld JL, Fonkalsrud EW, Coran AG, editors. Pediatric surgery. 5th ed. St Louis: Mosby Press; 1998. p. 1159–72.

Stringer MD, Oldham KT, Moriguard PDE. Pediatric surgery and urology. 2nd ed. Cambridge: Cambridge University Press; 2006. ISBN 9780521839020.

Shah SR, Gittes GK, Barsness KA, Kane TD. Multimedia article. Thoracoscopic patch repair of a right-sided congenital diaphragmatic hernia in a neonate. Surg Endosc. 2009;23(1):215.

Zwaveling S, van der Zee DC. Laparoscopic repair of an isolated congenital bilateral lumbar hernia in an infant. Eur J Pediatr Surg. 2012;22(4):321–3.

Holschneider AM, Hutson JM. Anorectal malformations in children: embryology, diagnosis, surgical treatment, follow-up. Berlin: Springer; 2006. ISBN 9783540317500.

Holschneider AM, Puri P. Hirschsprung's disease and allied disorders. Dordrecht: Springer; 2007. ISBN 9783540339342.

Ieiri S, Higashi M, Teshiba R, Saeki I, Esumi G, Akiyoshi J, Nakatsuji T, Taguchi T. Clinical features of Hirschsprung's disease associated with Down syndrome: a 30 year retrospective nationwide survey in Japan. J Pediatr Surg. 2009;44(12):2347–51.

Levitt MA, Peña A. Operative management of anomalies in female. In: Holschneider AM, Hutson J, editors. Anorectal malformations in children. Heidelberg: Springer; 2006a. p. 303–6.

Levitt MA, Peña A. Treatment of cloacas. In: Holschneider AM, Hutson J, editors. Anorectal malformations in children. Heidelberg: Springer; 2006b. p. 307–14.

Levitt MA, Pena A. Anorectal malformations. Rev Orphanet J Rare Dis. 2007; 2:33. doi:10.1186/1750-1172-2-33.

Nievelstein RA, Vos A, Valk J. MR imaging of anorectal malformations and associated anomalies. Eur Radiol. 1998;8(4):573–81.

Pena A, Levitt MA, Hong A, Midulla P. Surgical management of cloacal malformations: a review of 339 patients. J Pediatr Surg. 2004;39(3):470–9.

Pena A, Migotto-Krieger M, Levitt MA. Colostomy in anorectal malformations: a procedure with serious but preventable complications. J Pediatr Surg. 2006;41(4):748–56. Discussion 748-56.

Tei E, Yamataka A, Segawa O, Kobayashi H, Lane GJ, Tobayama S, Kameoka S, Miyano T. Laparoscopically assisted anorectovaginoplasty for selected types of female anorectal malformations. J Pediatr Surg. 2003;38(12):1770–4.

Teitelbaum DH, Coran AG, Weitzman JJ, Ziegler MM, Kane T. Hirschsprung's disease and related neuromuscular disorders of the intestine, Ch 94. In: O'Neill Jr JA, Rowe MI, Grosfeld JL,

Fonkalsrud EW, Coran AG, editors. Pediatric surgery. 5th ed. St Louis: Mosby Press; 1998. p. 1391–3.

Barsness KA, St Peter SD, Holcomb 3rd GW, Ostlie DJ, Kane TD. Laparoscopic fundoplication after previous open abdominal operations in infants and children. J Laparoendosc Adv Surg Tech A. 2009;19 Suppl 1:S47–9. 2009 Apr.

Lopez M, Kalfa N, Forgues D, Guibal MP, Galifer RB, Allal H. Laparoscopic redo fundoplication in children: failure causes and feasibility. J Pediatr Surg. 2008;43(10):1885–90.

Mauritz FA, van Herwaarden-Lindeboom MY, Stomp W, Zwaveling S, Fischer K, Houwen RH, Siersema PD, van der Zee DC. The effects and efficacy of antireflux surgery in children with gastroesophageal reflux disease: a systematic review. J Gastrointest Surg. 2011;15(10): 1872–8.

Rothenberg SS, Chin A. Laparoscopic Collis-Nissen for recurrent severe reflux in pediatric patients with esophageal atresia and recurrent hiatal hernia. J Laparoendosc Adv Surg Tech. 2010;20:787–90.

Tovar JA, Luis AL, Encinas JL, Burgos L, Pederiva F, Martinez L, Olivares P. Pediatric surgeons and gastroesophageal reflux. J Pediatr Surg. 2007;42(2):277–83.

Treef W, Schier F. Characteristics of laparoscopic inguinal hernia recurrences. Pediatr Surg Int. 2009;25(2):149–52.

Fraser JD, Ponsky TA, Aguayo P, Boulanger S, Parry R, Nixdorf N, DiLuciano J, Smith P, Sharp SW, Holcomb GW, Ostlie DJ, St Peter SD. Short-term natural history of the standard approaches for gastrostomy tube placement in the pediatric patient. J Laparoendosc Adv Surg Tech A. 2009;19(4):567–9.

Naiditch JA, Lautz T, Barsness KA. Postoperative complications in children undergoing gastrostomy tube placement. J Laparoendosc Adv Surg Tech. 2010;20:781–5.

Virnig DJ, Frech EJ, Delegge MH, Fang JC. Direct percutaneous endoscopic jejunostomy: a case series in pediatric patients. Gastrointest Endosc. 2008;67(6):984–7.

Coventry BJ, Watson DI, Tucker K, Chatterton B, Suppiah R. Intraoperative scintigraphic localization and laparoscopic excision of accessory splenic tissue. Surg Endosc. 1998;12(2):159–61.

Kollias J, Watson DI, Coventry BJ, Malycha P. Laparoscopic splenectomy using the lateral position: an improved technique. Aust N Z J Surg. 1995;65(10):746–8.

Watson DI, Coventry BJ, Chin T, Gill PG, Malycha P. Laparoscopic versus open splenectomy for immune thrombocytopenic purpura. Surgery. 1997;121(1):18–22.

# Chapter 4
# Pediatric Tumor Surgery

Anthony L. Sparnon and Brendon J. Coventry

## General Perspective and Overview

The relative risks and complications increase proportionately according to the site, size, and type and complexity of the problem being addressed within the chest and in relation to the age of the patient and other comorbidities. This is principally related to the surgical accessibility, ability to resect, risk of lung injury and respiratory compromise, functional reserve, technical ease, and the ability to achieve correction of the problem.

The main serious complications are **bleeding and infection,** which can be minimized by the adequate exposure, mobilization, technical care, and avoiding lung injury and hematoma formation. Infection is the main sequel of tissue injury, respiratory obstruction, and hematoma formation and may arise from preexisting infection or be newly acquired. This can lead to **pleural infection, lung consolidation, abdominal sepsis, abscess formation,** and **systemic sepsis. Multisystem failure** and **death** remain serious potential complications from surgery and systemic infection.

**Positioning on the operating table** has been associated with increased risk of **deep venous thrombosis** and **nerve palsies,** especially in prolonged procedures. **Limb ischemia, compartment syndrome,** and **ulnar** and **common peroneal nerve palsy** are recognized potential complications, which should be checked for, as the patient's position may change during surgery.

**Mortality** associated with most major surgical procedures is usually low and principally associated with infection or thromboembolism. Procedures involving the

A.L. Sparnon, MBBS, FRACS (✉)
Women's and Children's Hospital, North Adelaide, Australia
e-mail: asparnon@tps.com.au

B.J. Coventry, BMBS, PhD, FRACS, FACS, FRSM
Discipline of Surgery, Royal Adelaide Hospital, University of Adelaide,
L5 Eleanor Harrald Building, North Terrace, 5000 Adelaide, SA, Australia
e-mail: brendon.coventry@adelaide.edu.au

B.J. Coventry (ed.), *Pediatric Surgery*, Surgery: Complications, Risks and Consequences,      119
DOI 10.1007/978-1-4471-5439-6_4, © Springer-Verlag London 2014

major vessels, vena cava, or larger arteries carry higher risks associated with possible serious bleeding and infection, including increased risk of mortality. Rare failure of stapling devices can cause catastrophic bleeding. In children, mortality may more relate to comorbidities, for example, from underlying congenital problems.

This chapter therefore attempts to draw together in one place the estimated overall frequencies of the complications associated with pediatric tumor procedures, based on information obtained from the literature and experience. Not all patients are at risk of the full range of listed complications. It must be individualized for each patient and their disease process but represents a guide and summary of the attendant risks, complications, and consequences.

With these factors and facts in mind, the information given in this chapter must be appropriately and discernibly interpreted and used.

**Important Note**

It should be emphasized that the risks and frequencies that are given here *represent derived figures*. These *figures are best estimates of relative frequencies across most institutions*, not merely the highest-performing ones, and as such are often representative of a number of studies, which include different patients with differing comorbidities and different surgeons. In addition, the risks of complications in lower- or higher-risk patients may lie outside these estimated ranges, and individual clinical judgment is required as to the expected risks communicated to the patient and staff or for other purposes. The range of risks is also derived from experience and the literature; while risks outside this range may exist, certain risks may be reduced or absent due to variations of procedures or surgical approaches. It is recognized that different patients, practitioners, institutions, regions, and countries may vary in their requirements and recommendations.

For complications related to other associated/additional surgery that may arise during pediatric tumor surgery, see the relevant volume and chapter.

# Surgery for Neuroblastoma

## *Description*

Neuroblastoma is one of the more common solid tumors in childhood. It arises during fetal or early postnatal life from sympathetic cells derived from the neural crest and can be found in the adrenal medulla, sympathetic ganglia, or within preaortic ganglia. It is a highly malignant progressive tumor and the outlook for most children with advanced disease remains dismal. However, spontaneous regression and tumor maturation may occur into a benign ganglioneuroma. The incidence of neuroblastoma is about 1 in 10,000 with more than half presenting <4 years of age and 95 % having presented by the age of 10. Most arise in the abdomen, with the adrenal being the most common site (50 %), with tumors arising in the mediastinum in about 10 % and pelvis in 6 %. Metastases occur frequently to bone, liver, and lung. The management is based on the restratification that takes into account not only the stage but also clinical and biological variables. Low-stage tumors with favorable biological profiles are managed by surgical excision alone, with aggressive chemotherapy used for those with a poor biological profile. The management of high-risk disease is usually not amenable to resection. These children undergo biopsy followed by aggressive high-dose chemotherapy, with responders undergoing surgical resection of residual primary tumor with subsequent radiation to the primary and metastatic tumor sites. The incision(s), extent of resection, and complications are largely determined by the location and extent of disease.

## Anatomical Points

Preoperative planning using CT and MRI scans is essential in determining the anatomical extent of the tumor and the involvement and displacement of adjacent organs. Relatively large transverse incisions are required depending on tumor size and required access. The sigmoid and descending colons are reflected and spleen, pancreas, and the stomach mobilized to enable full access to the tumor. Initially, all major relevant vessels involved in the tumor should be completely displayed. Neuroblastoma does not usually invade the tunica media of major blood vessels and a plane of dissection may be developed between the tunica adventitia and tunic media.

## Perspective

See Table 4.1. The extent of disease dictates the extent of surgery and associated type and risk of complications. The dissection required to remove neuroblastoma is extremely tedious and time consuming with complications related specifically to the site of tumor and the respective vessels/organs involved. Extensive surgery is associated with a higher rate of complications and notably major complications. Injuries to major vessels, including the aorta, vena cava, and renal and mesenteric vessels, can result in major vascular complications with a significant operative mortality. Severe bleeding and injury to adjacent structures cause the most common immediate devastating problems that lead to immediate and further major complications such as infection, peritonitis, and abscess formation. Renal loss due to involvement with tumor, arterial damage, or renal vein thrombosis is a common complication. It is common to identify substantial lymphatic leakage during the course of surgery, and chylous ascites in the immediate postoperative period is frequently seen. This usually resolves within a week, but may persist causing severe distension. The insertion of peritoneovenous shunt may be required when the large collection persists and becomes symptomatic. Postoperative diarrhea is common in the initial postoperative period probably due to the dissection of the celiac and superior mesenteric arteries with damage to the inhibitory sympathetic nerve supply. This usually settles but may persist, producing

**Table 4.1** Surgery for neuroblastoma estimated frequency of complications, risks, and consequences

| Complications, risks, and consequences | Estimated frequency |
|---|---|
| ***Most significant/serious complications*** | |
| Mortality[a] | 1–5 % |
| Failure to remove tumor[a] | 1–5 % |
| Infection[b] | |
|   Subcutaneous | 1–5 % |
|   Wound | 1–5 % |
|   Intra-abdominal | 1–5 % |
|   Late postsplenectomy pneumonia/sepsis (with vaccination) | 0.1–1 % |
|   Chest infection | 1–5 % |
| Bleeding/laceration to aorta, inferior vena cava, mesenteric vessels, and renal vessels[b] | 1–5 % |
| Pancreatic injury/pancreatitis/pancreatic cyst/leakage/pancreatic fistula[a] | 1–5 % |
| Bowel injury (stomach, duodenum, small bowel, colon)[a] | 1–5 % |
| Radiation-induced enteritis[b] | 5–20 % |
| Renal/adrenal injury (incl. contralateral)[b] | 1–10 % |
| Seroma, lymphocele formation/lymph ascites/fistula[a] | |
|   Immediate | 20–50 % |
|   Prolonged | 1–5 % |
| Small bowel obstruction (early or late)[b] | 1–5 % |
| Potency, ejaculation problems in males[a] | 5–20 % |
| Splenic injury[b] | 1–5 % |
| Splenic conservation after injury[c] | |
|   Prolonged convalescence period | 50–80 % |
|   Limitation to activity | 50–80 % |
|   Late rupture | 0.1–1 % |
| Postoperative diarrhea[b] | 5–20 % |
| Neurological complications (with pelvic tumors)[a] (sciatic nerve palsy, neuropathic bladder, leg weakness) | 5–20 % |
| ***Rare significant/serious problems*** | |
| Hematoma formation[a] | 0.1–1 % |
| Bladder injury[a] | 0.1–1 % |
| Diaphragmatic injury[a] | 0.1–1 % |
| Subphrenic abscess[a] | 0.1–1 % |
| Stoma formation[a] | 0.1–1 % |
| Nerve injury (lumbar plexus or branches, sympathetic chain)[b] | 0.1–1 % |
| ***Less serious complications*** | |
| Pain/discomfort/tenderness | |
|   Short term (<4 weeks) | 20–50 % |
|   Longer term (>12 weeks) | 0.1–1 % |
| Paralytic ileus[a] | 20–50 % |
| Sensory changes | <0.1 % |
| Urinary retention/catheterization[b] | 0.1–1 % |
| Wound scarring (deformity/dimpling of wound scar/poor cosmesis) | 1–5 % |
| Drain tube(s)[b] | 5–20 % |

[a]Incidence may be higher for moderate and massive tumors; stomas carry additional risks
[b]Dependent on underlying pathology, surgical technique, preferences, comorbidities, and location
[c]Splenic preservation may sometimes be possible for splenic traumatic injury

problems in the long-term survivors. Injury to the pancreas can result in pancreatic leakage with collections, pancreatitis, infections, and external fistulae. Small bowel obstruction due to adhesions is relatively infrequent but may occur after extensive operative dissection and associated radiotherapy. Management may require major surgery. Pelvic neuroblastoma is associated with a significant incidence of neurological problems including sciatic nerve palsy, urinary and fecal incontinence, neuropathic bladder, and leg weakness. Death occurs in a significant number due to the major associated vascular injuries, splenic damage, and associated metabolic problems.

## *Major Complications/Consequences*

Early **death** is usually related to catastrophic **bleeding** or early postoperative **infection** leading to **abscess formation, systemic sepsis,** and **multisystem organ failure.** Late mortality is due to **tumor recurrence. Renal loss** is common in children with compromised renal function following chemotherapy. **Bowel injury** is often associated with ischemia and can be debilitating, especially in a child who has had radiotherapy. Significant lymphatic leakage from thoracic duct injury resulting in **lymphatic or chylous ascites** can be debilitating. **Pancreatic leakage, persistent collections, and fistulas** while rare can require surgical intervention. **Small bowel obstruction** can be a recurrent major issue requiring **repeated surgery,** carrying considerable risk. Despite risk of numerous complications, complete excision of neuroblastoma may confer a survival advantage and outweigh the conservative approach. As with most complex surgery, these risks need to be evaluated carefully for the individual and balanced accordingly.

---

**Consent and Risk Reduction**

**Main Points to Explain**

- GA risk
- Pain/discomfort
- Bleeding/hematoma*
- Infection (local/systemic)*
- Urinary obstruction*
- Urine leakage*
- Urine collection*
- Risk of other abdominal organ injury*
- Possible stoma formation*
- Possible blood transfusion
- Possible tumor recurrence*
- Possible further surgery*
- Risks without surgery*

   ***Dependent on pathology, comorbidities, and surgery performed**

---

# Further Reading, References, and Resources

Azizkhan RG et al. Surgical complications of neuroblastoma resection. Surgery. 1985;97(5):514–7.

Canete A et al. Surgical treatment for neuroblastoma: complications during 15 years experience. J Pediatr Surg. 1999;33(10):1526–30.

Cruccetti A, Kiely EM, Spitz L, Drake DP, Pritchard J, Pierro A. Pelvic neuroblastoma: low mortality and high morbidity. J Pediatr Surg. 2000;35(5):724–8.

Fraga JC, Rothenberg S, Kiely E, Pierro A. Video-assisted thoracic surgery resection for pediatric mediastinal neurogenic tumors. J Pediatr Surg. 2012;47(7):1349–53.

Kiely E. A technique for excision of abdominal and pelvic neuroblastoma. Ann R Coll Surg Engl. 2007;89(4):342–48.

Koivusalo AI, Pakarinen MP, Rintala RJ, Saarinen-Pihkala UM. Surgical treatment of neuroblastoma: twenty-three years of experience at a single institution. Surg Today. 2013; 12 Apr 2013. (Epub ahead of print).

Kubota M et al. Long-term follow up status of patients with neuroblastoma after undergoing either aggressive surgery or chemotherapy – a single institutional experience. J Pediatr Surg. 2004; 39(9):1328–32.

Moon SB, Park KW, Jung SE, Youn WJ. Neuroblastoma: treatment outcome after incomplete resection of primary tumors. Pediatr Surg Int. 2009;25(9):789–93.

Zwaveling S, Tytgat GA, van der Zee DC, Wijnen MH, Heij HA. Is complete surgical resection of stage 4 neuroblastoma a prerequisite for optimal survival or may >95 % tumour resection suffice? Pediatr Surg Int. 2012;28(10):953–9.

# Chapter 5
# Thoracic Surgery

Christopher Kirby, John Hutson, Jayme Bennetts,
and Brendon J. Coventry

## General Perspective and Overview

The relative risks and complications increase proportionately according to the site, size, and type and complexity of the problem being addressed within the chest and in relation to the age of the patient and other comorbidities. This is principally related to the surgical accessibility, ability to resect, risk of lung injury and respiratory compromise, functional reserve, technical ease, and the ability to achieve correction of the problem.

The main serious complications are **bleeding and infection,** which can be minimized by the adequate exposure, mobilization, technical care, and avoiding lung injury and hematoma formation. Infection is the main sequel of tissue injury, respiratory obstruction, and hematoma formation and may arise from preexisting infection or be newly acquired. This can lead to **pleural infection, lung consolidation, abscess formation,** and **systemic sepsis. Multisystem failure** and **death** remain serious potential complications from thoracic surgery and systemic infection.

C. Kirby, FRCS, FRACS
Department of Paediatric Surgery, Women's and Children's
Hospital, Adelaide, Australia

J. Hutson, BS, MD, FRACS, DSc, FRAP (hon)
Department of Paediatrics, Royal Children's Hospital,
Melbourne, Australia

J. Bennetts, BMBS, FRACS, FCSANZ
Cardiac and Thoracic Surgery, Flinders Medical Centre,
Adelaide, Australia

B.J. Coventry, BMBS, PhD, FRACS, FACS, FRSM (✉)
Discipline of Surgery, Royal Adelaide Hospital, University of Adelaide,
L5 Eleanor Harrald Building, North Terrace, 5000 Adelaide, SA, Australia
e-mail: brendon.coventry@adelaide.edu.au

B.J. Coventry (ed.), *Pediatric Surgery*, Surgery: Complications, Risks and Consequences,     125
DOI 10.1007/978-1-4471-5439-6_5, © Springer-Verlag London 2014

**Neural injuries** are not infrequent potential problems associated with thoracic surgery and access, because intercostal nerves travel beneath each rib and may be involved in direct incision, compression from retractors, or scar formation.

**Positioning on the operating table** has been associated with increased risk of **deep venous thrombosis** and **nerve palsies**, especially in prolonged procedures. **Limb ischemia, compartment syndrome, and ulnar** and **common peroneal nerve palsy** are recognized potential complications, which should be checked for, as the patient's position may change during surgery.

**Mortality** associated with most thoracic surgery procedures is usually low and principally associated with pulmonary infarction or thromboembolism. Procedures involving the pulmonary vessels, vena cava, or larger arteries carry higher risks associated with possible serious bleeding and infection, including increased risk of mortality. Rare failure of stapling devices can cause catastrophic bleeding. In children, mortality may more relate to comorbidities, for example, from underlying congenital problems.

This chapter therefore attempts to draw together in one place the estimated overall frequencies of the complications associated with thoracic procedures, based on information obtained from the literature and experience. Not all patients are at risk of the full range of listed complications. It must be individualized for each patient and their disease process but represents a guide and summary of the attendant risks, complications, and consequences.

With these factors and facts in mind, the information given in this chapter must be appropriately and discernibly interpreted and used.

---

**Important Note**

It should be emphasized that the risks and frequencies that are given here *represent derived figures*. These *figures are best estimates of relative frequencies across most institutions*, not merely the highest-performing ones, and as such are often representative of a number of studies, which include different patients with differing comorbidities and different surgeons. In addition, the risks of complications in lower- or higher-risk patients may lie outside these estimated ranges, and individual clinical judgment is required as to the expected risks communicated to the patient and staff or for other purposes. The range of risks is also derived from experience and the literature; while risks outside this range may exist, certain risks may be reduced or absent due to variations of procedures or surgical approaches. It is recognized that different patients, practitioners, institutions, regions, and countries may vary in their requirements and recommendations.

---

For complications related to other associated/additional surgery that may arise during thoracic surgery, see Volume 4 Esophageal Surgery or Chap. 8 of Volume 6 Cardiac Surgery or the relevant volume and chapter.

## Acknowledgments

The authors would like to thank Dr. Warwick Teague, Adelaide, Australia, for reviewing parts of the manuscript and Dr. Craig Jurisevic for some of the adult thoracic surgery information.

## Bronchoscopy and/or Extraction of Respiratory Foreign Bodies

### Description

General anesthesia is typically used. Video-assisted flexible bronchoscopy is a minimally invasive approach to visualization of the respiratory tract. Rigid bronchoscopy may be used in some situations and some thoracic surgeons prefer this method. Either method involves the insertion of a bronchoscope down the airways to examine, biopsy, wash out (lavage), or remove foreign material. Aspiration of a foreign body remains a very common pediatric emergency problem. The risk of injury is increased with the use of rigid versus flexible bronchoscopes, but in experienced hands the risks are very small.

### Anatomical Points

The anatomy of the bronchial tree is relatively constant, and the procedures are more affected by the chest wall shape, jaw movement, oral cavity shape, and neck mobility. The right main-stem bronchus is in a straighter line with the trachea than the left, and so foreign material from aspiration more often enters the right side. The position of the foreign material, defect, or neoplasm can be critical in determining the ease and relative safety of the procedure.

### Perspective

See Table 5.1. Bronchoscopy by any method is usually associated with few, if any, complications. Oral lacerations and teeth fractures can be significant complications, but lacerations or bruising of mucosa are usually minor. These are often avoidable with careful attention and teeth guards. Serious complications are relatively rare. These include bleeding, worsening of infection, laceration of the airway, and very rarely airway rupture, which may be small and self-limiting or large with a persistent air leak associated with mediastinal gas, mediastinitis, and even pneumothorax.

**Table 5.1** Bronchoscopy including removal of respiratory foreign bodies estimated frequency of complications, risks, and consequences

| Complications, risks, and consequences | Estimated frequency |
|---|---|
| Oral/airway injury[a] | 1–5 % |
| Bleeding (minor) | 5–20 % |
| *Rare significant/serious problems* | |
| Bleeding (major) | 0.1–1 % |
| Infection | |
|   Subcutaneous/wound | 0.1–1 % |
|   Intrathoracic (pneumonia, pleural) | 0.1–1 % |
|   Mediastinitis | 0.1–1 % |
|   Systemic | 0.1–1 % |
| Teeth fracture[a] | 0.1–1 % |
| Pulmonary injury (direct or indirect)[a] | 0.1–1 % |
| Arrhythmias | 0.1–1 % |
| Thoracoscopy or thoracotomy (failed removal)[a] | 0.1–1 % |
| Airway stenosis[a] | 0.1–1 % |
| Surgical emphysema | <0.1 % |
| Hematoma formation | |
|   Retropharyngeal | <0.1 % |
| Pleural drain tube(s)[a] | <0.1 % |

[a]Dependent on underlying anatomy, pathology, location of disease, and/or surgical preference

## Major Complications

The most serious complication of the bronchoscopic approach to intrathoracic pathology is **airway rupture**, which is very rare. **Mediastinal air**, **mediastinitis**, **pneumothorax**, or **persistent air leak** may result. **Thoracotomy** may then be required. **Worsening of infection** is not uncommon in those with existing serious airway infection. Mucosal injury can cause **bleeding** which can be significant especially in the anticoagulated patient. This can usually be controlled with cautery. **Airway collapse**, **basal atelectasis**, and sometimes secondary **lung infection** are uncommon and may affect either lung. **Empyema** and **abscess formation** are very rare but are severe if they occur leading to prolonged hospital stay and other sequelae. **Multisystem organ failure** is extremely rare and serious, the incidence being most related to the underlying lung pathology and other comorbidities.

**Consent and Risk Reduction**

**Main Points to Explain**

- Discomfort
- Oral/teeth/neck injury
- Airway Injury
- Pneumonia
- Pneumothorax (rare)
- Cardiac arrhythmias (usually minor)
- Further surgery

## Diagnostic Thoracoscopy Including Video-Assisted Thoracoscopy

### Description

General anesthesia is used. Video-assisted thoracoscopy is a minimally invasive approach to intrathoracic surgical conditions and is being increasingly used. It involves the formation of several (usually 2–3) thoracoscopy ports. This involves creating 0.5–1-cm skin incisions, with dissection through the intercostal spaces and, thus, into the pleural space. The exact location of these thoracoscopy ports is dictated by the intrathoracic problem in question. For pulmonary parenchymal resections (e.g., lung biopsies), two 1-cm ports are made in the 5th intercostal space, the first in the anterior axillary line and the second in the midaxillary line. A further 5-mm port is made in the 4th intercostal space in the posterior axillary line. These port placements can also be used for resection of anterior mediastinal lesions such as germ cell tumors or thymic masses. To approach the posterior mediastinum, the ports must be made in the 3rd, 4th, and 6th intercostal spaces in a vertical line in a position between the midaxillary and anterior axillary lines. Pleural conditions requiring resection or biopsy can be approached simply by two ports in the 6th or 7th intercostal space between the midaxillary and anterior axillary lines. These ports are placed in a lower intercostal space than for pulmonary or mediastinal lesions, such that drains can be placed in a more dependent position to allow more complete drainage of pleural fluid (e.g., to allow for an effective pleurodesis in malignant effusions).

### Anatomical Points

The abovementioned thoracoscopy sites may have to be varied depending on the position of the lesion to be inspected, biopsied, or resected. In particular, lower lobe pulmonary parenchymal lesions often necessitate the use of ports placed in the 6th or 7th intercostal spaces. Pleural adhesions are not uncommon and may prevent successful thoracoscopic surgery. If the pleural space is obliterated, then thoracoscopy will be impossible and the surgeon would need to resort to open thoracotomy. With a partially obliterated pleural space, pleural adhesions can be dissected and allow enough mobilization of the lung to permit the procedure to be carried out thoracoscopically.

### Perspective

See Table 5.2. A significant number of intrathoracic surgical procedures are now performed using the thoracoscopic approach. The main limitation of the thoracoscopic approach involves the fact that, by virtue of the inability to palpate intrathoracic organs, small pulmonary parenchymal lesions not evident on visual inspection of the lung alone may be difficult to locate and thus resect. Serious complications are relatively rare.

**Table 5.2** Diagnostic thoracoscopy estimated frequency of complications, risks, and consequences

| Complications, risks, and consequences | Estimated frequency |
|---|---|
| *Most significant/serious complications* | |
| Infection | |
|    Subcutaneous/wound | 1–5 % |
|    Intrathoracic (pneumonia, pleural) | 1–5 % |
|    Mediastinitis | 0.1–1 % |
|    Systemic | 0.1–1 % |
| Pneumothorax (residual) | 1–5 % |
| *Rare significant/serious problems* | |
| Pulmonary empyema | 0.1–1 % |
| Pulmonary abscess | 0.1–1 % |
| Bleeding | 0.1–1 % |
| Hematoma formation | |
|    Wound | 0.1–1 % |
|    Hemothorax | 0.1–1 % |
|    Pulmonary contusion | 0.1–1 % |
| Recurrent laryngeal nerve injury | 0.1–1 % |
| Surgical emphysema | 0.1–1 % |
| Persistent air leak | 0.1–1 % |
| Bronchopleural fistula | 0.1–1 % |
| Arrhythmias | 0.1–1 % |
| Pericardial effusion | 0.1–1 % |
| Myocardial injury, cardiac failure, MI (hypotension) | 0.1–1 % |
| Pulmonary injury (direct or inferior pulmonary vein injury) | 0.1–1 % |
| Diaphragmatic injury paresis (including phrenic nerve injury)[a] | <0.1 % |
| Diaphragmatic hernia | <0.1 % |
| Thoracic duct injury (chylous leak, fistula) | <0.1 % |
| Multisystem failure (renal, pulmonary, cardiac failure)[a] | 0.1–1 % |
| Venous thrombosis | 0.1–1 % |
| Mortality | |
| Mortality <u>without</u> surgery | |
| *Less serious complications* | |
| Pain/tenderness [rib pain, wound pain] | |
|    Acute (<4weeks) | 50–80 % |
|    Chronic (>12weeks) | 0.1–1 % |
| Wound scarring or port site or minithoracotomy | 1–5 % |
| Deformity of rib or skin (poor cosmesis) | 1–5 % |
| Pleural drain tube(s)[a] | 50–80 % |

[a]Dependent on underlying anatomy, pathology, location of disease, and/or surgical preference

## Major Complications

The most serious complication of the thoracoscopic approach to intrathoracic pathology is **bleeding** from the intercostal vessels. This can usually be controlled through the thoracoscopy port but, rarely, will require a **minithoracotomy** (in the same intercostal space) to control the bleeding. **Intercostal neuralgia** can occur following thoracoscopy but is significantly less frequent than following thoracotomy.

Inadvertent **injury to the lung** is also possible especially in the presence of dense pleural adhesions, and occasionally **pneumothorax** or **persistent air leak** may result. Complications specific to the underlying problem and reason for the thoracoscopy may occur. **Basal atelectasis** and sometimes secondary **lung infection** are not uncommon and may affect either lung. **Empyema** and **abscess formation** are very rare but are severe if they occur leading to prolonged hospital stay and other sequelae. **Multisystem organ failure** is extremely serious, the incidence being most related to the underlying lung pathology and other comorbidities.

---

**Consent and Risk Reduction**

**Main Points to Explain**

- Discomfort
- Bruising and bleeding
- Infection
- Persistent pneumothorax (rare)
- Cardiac arrhythmias (usually minor)
- Failure of insertion/resection
- Further surgery

---

# Thoracotomy (Lateral Intercostal or Median Sternotomy)

## *Description*

General anesthesia is used. Thoracotomy involves a full-thickness incision into the pleural space by way of the intercostal space. A thoracotomy can be anterolateral, lateral, posterolateral, or manubriosternal depending on the intrathoracic pathology being attended to. Thoracotomy alone is typically used for exploration, diagnosis, biopsy, decortication, pleurodesis, and the like.

An *anterolateral thoracotomy* involves an incision between the midclavicular line and the anterior axillary line, usually through the 5th intercostal space.

A true *lateral thoracotomy* involves an incision situated between the anterior and posterior lines in the 5th or 6th intercostal space incising through serratus anterior and the anterior border of the latissimus dorsi muscles.

A *posterolateral thoracotomy* involves extension of the lateral thoracotomy skin incision below the tip of the scapular and extending posterosuperiorly between the medial border of the scapular and the vertebral spinous processes. The incision extends through serratus anterior muscle and latissimus dorsi and can also extend to involve the trapezius and paraspinal group of muscles.

An *anterior thoracotomy* involves dissection through the serratus anterior muscle and the intercostal muscle.

Once the intercostal muscles and parietal pleura have been dissected, then a retractor is placed between the ribs and opened. To facilitate the opening of the intercostal space, a short segment of the posterior rib (either above or below) can be resected, but children usually have very flexible ribs.

A *median sternotomy* involves a skin incision located between the suprasternal notch and the xiphisternum. A midline division of the manubrium, sternal body, and xiphisternal process is then performed, using a bone saw. This incision allows access to the pericardium and medial aspect of both pleural spaces.

## Anatomical Points

There are few anatomical variants that affect this procedure; however, chest wall deformities such as pectus excavatum and scoliosis may alter the ease of approach and therefore the complications. Acquired anatomical changes due to disease, including trauma or previous surgery, can also affect the ease and results of surgery.

## Perspective

See Table 5.3. The various thoracotomy incisions require significant muscle dissection and result in trauma to the ribs and costovertebral, costotransverse, costochondral, and sternochondral joints. Thus, postoperative pain is a significant issue. Furthermore, dissection of the parietal pleura and the introduction of air and blood into the pleural space result in a pleuritic response, which contributes significantly to the patient's overall pain. Postoperative analgesia in the thoracotomy patient is significantly improved with the use of thoracic epidural catheters and paravertebral (extrapleural) catheters through which analgesia can be administered.

## Major Complications

The major complication directly related to a thoracotomy approach is **bleeding**, either from the chest wall musculature or the intercostal vessels. **Intercostal neuralgia**, secondary to intercostal nerve injury and/or scarring, occurs more frequently than in thoracoscopic procedures and can be permanent in some cases.

**Costochondritis** can occur secondary to trauma at the costochondral joints. This may occur not only in the intercostal space involved but also in costochondral joints several ribs above and below the incisions. Inadvertent **injury to the lung** is also possible especially in the presence of dense pleural adhesions, and occasionally **pneumothorax** or **persistent air leak** may result. Complications specific to the

**Table 5.3** Thoracotomy estimated frequency of complications, risks, and consequences

| Complications, risks, and consequences | Estimated frequency |
|---|---|
| *Most significant/serious complications* | |
| Infection | |
|   Subcutaneous/wound | 1–5 % |
|   Intrathoracic (pneumonia, pleural) | 1–5 % |
|   Mediastinitis | 0.1–1 % |
|   Systemic | 0.1–1 % |
| Pneumothorax | 1–5 % |
| *Rare significant/serious problems* | |
| Pulmonary empyema | 0.1–1 % |
| Pulmonary abscess | 0.1–1 % |
| Bleeding | 0.1–1 % |
| Hematoma formation | |
|   Wound | 0.1–1 % |
|   Hemothorax | 0.1–1 % |
|   Pulmonary contusion | 0.1–1 % |
| Recurrent laryngeal nerve injury | 0.1–1 % |
| Persistent air leak | 0.1–1 % |
| Bronchopleural fistula | 0.1–1 % |
| Arrhythmias | 0.1–1 % |
| Pericardial effusion | 0.1–1 % |
| Myocardial injury, cardiac failure, MI (hypotension) | 0.1–1 % |
| Pulmonary injury (direct or inferior pulmonary vein injury) | 0.1–1 % |
| Multisystem failure (renal, pulmonary, cardiac failure)[a] | 0.1–1 % |
| Venous thrombosis | 0.1–1 % |
| Sternal wire protrusion/erosion/pain (if median sternotomy used)[a] | 0.1–1 % |
| Diaphragmatic injury paresis | <0.1 % |
| Thoracic duct injury (chylous leak, fistula) | <0.1 % |
| Osteomyelitis of ribs[a] | <0.1 % |
| *For malignancy* | |
| Unresectability of malignancy/involved resection margins[a] | 1–5 % |
| Recurrence/progressive disease[a] | 1–5 % |
| *Including surgery through the diaphragm* | |
| Liver injury/bowel Injury/pancreatitis | 0.1–1 % |
| Splenic injury | 0.1–1 % |
|   Conservation (consequent limitation to activity, late rupture) | 0.1–1 % |
|   Splenectomy | 0.1–1 % |
| Diaphragmatic hernia | <0.1 % |
| Mortality | |
| Mortality <u>without</u> surgery | |
| *Less serious complications* | |
| Pain/tenderness [rib pain, wound pain] | |
|   Acute (<4weeks) | >80 % |
|   Chronic (>12weeks) | 1–5 % |
| Surgical emphysema | 0.1–1 % |

(continued)

**Table 5.3** (continued)

| Complications, risks, and consequences | Estimated frequency |
|---|---|
| Wound scarring | 5–20 |
| Deformity of rib/chest or skin (poor cosmesis) | 1–5 |
| Pleural drain tube(s)[a] | 50–80 |

Note: When a thoracotomy includes esophageal or paraesophageal or esophagogastric surgery, it is associated with the risks, consequences, and complications of those additional procedures, and when a thoracotomy is combined with a laparotomy (thoracolaparotomy), the risks, consequences, and complications of laparotomy should also be included

[a]Dependent on underlying pathology, location of disease, and/or surgical preference

underlying problem and reason for the thoracotomy may occur. **Basal atelectasis** and sometimes secondary **lung infection** are not uncommon and may affect either lung. **Empyema** and **abscess formation** are very rare but are severe if they occur leading to prolonged hospital stay and other sequelae. **Multisystem organ failure** is extremely serious, the incidence being most related to the underlying lung pathology and other comorbidities.

---

**Consent and Risk Reduction**

**Main Points to Explain**

- Discomfort/pain
- Bruising and bleeding
- Infection
- Persistent pneumothorax (rare)
- Cardiac arrhythmias (usually minor)
- Failure of access
- Further surgery
- MSOF and death

---

## Partial Lung Resection

### *Description*

General anesthesia is used. A partial lung resection may take the form of a wedge resection, segmental resection, single lobectomy, or bi-lobectomy, greatly facilitated by the use of lung stapling devices. A *wedge resection* involves a non-anatomical resection of a portion of the lung, most commonly for resection of peripheral lung nodules, where the lesion of interest is resected with a small amount of surrounding lung tissue in the shape of a wedge. A *segmental resection* (or segmentectomy) involves resection of the anatomical segment including segmental bronchus arteries and veins and segmental lymph nodes. A *lobectomy* is an anatomical resection of the entire lobe, which includes the lobar pulmonary arterial and venous supply and accompanying lobar lymph nodes. The interlobar fissures (oblique and horizontal on the right and oblique on the left) are commonly incomplete. The fissures can be completed using standard pulmonary stapling devices.

## *Anatomical Points*

Chest wall deformities such as pectus excavatum and scoliosis may alter the ease of approach and therefore the complications. Acquired anatomical changes due to disease, including trauma or previous surgery, can also affect the ease and results of surgery. Fusion of some of the lung fissures may occur making the dissection more difficult. The most common *pulmonary vascular* variation involves the pulmonary venous supply. In 10 % of patients the right middle lobe pulmonary vein drains directly into the inferior pulmonary vein rather than the superior pulmonary vein. In 2–5 % of patients, there may be a single pulmonary vein receiving tributaries from all lobes. The lobar pulmonary arterial and venous supply is very variable, thus necessitating careful dissection and identification of individual lobar and segmental vessels prior to ligation and transection. Anatomical variation of the *bronchial tree* is much less common than that of vascular supply. The intra- and extra-pericardial courses of the pulmonary vessels are quite variable, often necessitating the opening of the pericardium for full assessment. This maneuver often allows the surgeon to fully assess the extent of involvement of the vessels by lesions occurring in a central (hilar, mediastinal) location.

## *Perspective*

See Table 5.4. The major debility resulting from partial lung resections (wedge resection, segmentectomy, or lobectomy) is **empyema** (pleural space infection). This occurs more commonly when, after resection, there is a significant residual air space. The other major debility resulting from partial lung resection is post-resection **bronchopleural fistula**. This occurs more commonly in patients with severe underlying lung disease and can result from a leaking bronchial stump or leakage from a pulmonary parenchymal staple line.

   **Chylothorax** can result from damage to the thoracic duct within the chest and occurs more commonly where there has been extensive mediastinal or esophageal dissection.

   **Intercostal neuralgia**, when it occurs, is usually temporary but may be permanent in some cases. More commonly there is a small area of anterior chest wall **numbness or paresthesia** in the distribution of the intercostal nerve traumatized at the time of thoracotomy.

**Table 5.4** Partial lung resection estimated frequency of complications, risks, and consequences

| Complications, risks, and consequences | Estimated frequency |
|---|---|
| ***Most significant/serious complications*** | |
| Infection | |
|   Subcutaneous/wound | 1–5 % |
|   Intrathoracic (pneumonia, pleural) | 1–5 % |
|   Mediastinitis | 0.1–1 % |
|   Systemic | 0.1–1 % |
| Pneumothorax | 1–5 % |
| Rib resection[a] | 20–50 % |
| ***Rare significant/serious problems*** | |
| Pulmonary empyema | 0.1–1 % |
| Pulmonary abscess | 0.1–1 % |
| Bleeding | 0.1–1 % |
| Hematoma formation | |
|   Wound | 0.1–1 % |
|   Hemothorax | 0.1–1 % |
|   Pulmonary contusion | 0.1–1 % |
| Surgical emphysema | 0.1–1 % |
| Persistent air leak[a] | 0.1–1 % |
| Bronchopleural fistula[a] | 0.1–1 % |
| Arrhythmias | 0.1–1 % |
| Pericardial effusion | 0.1–1 % |
| Myocardial injury, cardiac failure, MI (hypotension) | 0.1–1 % |
| Pulmonary injury (direct or inferior pulmonary vein injury) | 0.1–1 % |
| Multi system failure (renal, pulmonary, cardiac failure)[a] | 0.1–1 % |
| Venous thrombosis | 0.1–1 % |
| Sternal wire protrusion/erosion/pain (if used)[a] | 0.1–1 % |
| Osteomyelitis of ribs[a] | <0.1 % |
| Diaphragmatic injury paresis | <0.1 % |
| Thoracic duct injury (chylous leak, fistula)[a] | <0.1 % |
| Recurrent laryngeal nerve injury | <0.1 % |
| *For malignancy* | |
| Unresectability of malignancy/involved resection margins[a] | 1–5 % |
| Recurrence/progressive disease[a] | 1–5 % |
| Mortality | |
| Mortality <u>without</u> surgery | |
| ***Less serious complications*** | |
| Pain/tenderness [rib pain, wound pain] | |
|   Acute (<4weeks) | >80 % |
|   Chronic (>12weeks) | 1–5 % |
| Wound scarring | 5–20 % |
| Deformity of rib/chest or skin (poor cosmesis) | 1–5 % |
| Pleural drain tube(s)[a] | 50–80 % |

[a]Dependent on underlying pathology, location of disease, and/or surgical preference

## *Major Complications*

The most serious complications are **empyema** and **abscess formation**. Many patients will require a surgical drainage procedure; with the consequential debility, this entails including prolonged hospital stay and other sequelae. Inadvertent **injury to the lung** is also possible especially in the presence of dense pleural adhesions, and occasionally **pneumothorax** or **persistent air leak** may result. Complications specific to the underlying problem and reason for the partial lung resection may occur. **Basal atelectasis** and sometimes secondary **lung infection** are not uncommon and may affect either lung. **Chylothorax** and **bronchopleural fistula** formation are chronic debilitating problems that delay recovery significantly. **Multisystem organ failure** is extremely serious, the incidence being most related to the underlying lung pathology and other comorbidities, and is associated with mortality.

---

**Consent and Risk Reduction**

**Main Points to Explain**

- Discomfort/pain
- Bruising and bleeding
- Infection
- Persistent pneumothorax (rare)
- Cardiac arrhythmias (usually minor)
- Failure of access/resection
- Further surgery
- MSOF and death

---

## Pneumonectomy

## *Description*

General anesthesia is used. A pneumonectomy is performed via a posterolateral thoracotomy. This procedure involves complete mobilization and isolation of the right or left pulmonary arteries and the superior and inferior pulmonary veins. It is often safer to divide the pulmonary veins prior to the artery since this may allow for more length and an easier division of the pulmonary artery. The main-stem bronchus is then divided as close to the carina as possible, and the bronchial stump may be buttressed with either a flap of pleura or an intercostal muscle flap. When a pneumonectomy is performed for bronchogenic carcinoma, mediastinal lymph node sampling is a standard part of the procedure.

## Anatomical Points

Chest wall deformities such as pectus excavatum and scoliosis may alter the ease of approach and therefore the complications. Acquired anatomical changes due to disease, including trauma or previous surgery, can also affect the ease and results of surgery. Fusion of some of the lung fissures may occur making the dissection more difficult. The most common *pulmonary vascular* variation involves the pulmonary venous supply. In 10 % of patients the right middle lobe pulmonary vein drains directly into the inferior pulmonary vein rather than the superior pulmonary vein. In 2–5 % of patients, there may be a single pulmonary vein receiving tributaries from all lobes. The lobar pulmonary arterial and venous supply is very variable, thus necessitating careful dissection and identification of individual lobar and segmental vessels prior to ligation and transection. Anatomical variation of the *bronchial tree* is much less common than that of vascular supply. The intra- and extra-pericardial courses of the pulmonary vessels are quite variable, often necessitating the opening of the pericardium for full assessment. This maneuver often allows the surgeon to fully assess the extent of involvement of the vessels by lesions occurring in a central (hilar; mediastinal) location.

## Perspective

See Table 5.5. Pleural space infection (**empyema**) is more common following pneumonectomy than partial lung resection. This is by virtue of the fact that there is a large residual air space. Fluid eventually fills the cavity. **Bronchopleural fistula** is also a significant problem and occurs more commonly on the right than left, due to the more exposed nature of the right main bronchus following pneumonectomy. The incidence of a bronchopleural fistula can be reduced by covering the bronchial stump with a pleural or intercostal muscle flap at the time of pneumonectomy. **Chylothorax** can result from damage to the thoracic duct within the chest and occurs more commonly where there has been extensive mediastinal dissection, for example, during a mediastinal lymph node clearance for bronchogenic carcinoma, or esophageal resection. **Intercostal neuralgia**, when it occurs, is usually temporary but may be permanent in some cases. More commonly there is a small area of anterior chest wall **numbness or paresthesia** in the distribution of the intercostal nerve traumatized at the time of thoracotomy.

## Major Complications

One of the most significant complications following pneumonectomy is **postpneumonectomy pulmonary edema** in the remaining lung. This occurs more commonly following a right pneumonectomy and results from the significantly increased postoperative pulmonary vascular resistance and subsequent cardiac compromise. This has a high

**Table 5.5**  Pneumonectomy estimated frequency of complications, risks, and consequences

| Complications, risks, and consequences | Estimated frequency |
|---|---|
| ***Most significant/serious complications*** | |
| Infection | |
|    Subcutaneous/wound | 1–5 % |
|    Intrathoracic (pneumonia, pleural) | 1–5 % |
|    Mediastinitis | 0.1–1 % |
|    Systemic | 0.1–1 % |
| Pneumothorax | 1–5 % |
| Pulmonary failure[a] | 1–5 % |
| Prolonged assisted ventilation[a] | 1–5 % |
| ***Rare significant/serious problems*** | |
| Pulmonary empyema | 0.1–1 % |
| Pulmonary abscess | 0.1–1 % |
| Bleeding | 0.1–1 % |
| Hematoma formation | |
|    Wound | 0.1–1 % |
|    Hemothorax | 0.1–1 % |
|    Pulmonary contusion | 0.1–1 % |
| Recurrent laryngeal nerve injury | 0.1–1 % |
| Surgical emphysema | 0.1–1 % |
| Persistent air leak[a] | 0.1–1 % |
| Bronchopleural fistula[a] | 0.1–1 % |
| Arrhythmias | 0.1–1 % |
| Pericardial effusion | 0.1–1 % |
| Myocardial injury, cardiac failure, MI (hypotension) | 0.1–1 % |
| Pulmonary injury (direct or inferior pulmonary vein injury) | 0.1–1 % |
| Esophageal injury[a] | 0.1–1 % |
| Multisystem failure (renal, pulmonary, cardiac failure)[a] | 0.1–1 % |
| Venous thrombosis | 0.1–1 % |
| Sternal wire protrusion/erosion/pain (if used, median sternotomy)[a] | 0.1–1 % |
| Diaphragmatic injury paresis | <0.1 % |
| Thoracic duct injury (chylous leak, fistula)[a] | <0.1 % |
| Osteomyelitis of ribs[a] | <0.1 % |
| Death[a] | 1–5 % |
| *For malignancy* | |
| Unresectability of malignancy/involved resection margins[a] | 1–5 % |
| Recurrence/progressive disease[a] | 1–5 % |
| Mortality | |
| Mortality <u>without</u> surgery | |
| ***Less serious complications*** | |
| Pain/tenderness [rib pain, wound pain] | |
|    Acute (<4weeks) | >80 % |
|    Chronic (>12weeks) | 1–5 % |
| Wound scarring | 5–20 % |
| Deformity of rib/chest or skin (poor cosmesis) | 1–5 % |
| Pleural drain tube(s)[a] | 50–80 % |

[a]Dependent on underlying pathology, location of disease, and/or surgical preference

mortality and is exceptionally difficult to treat. Fluid restriction postpneumonectomy is successful in reducing the incidence of this complication. Another significant complication particularly following left pneumonectomy is that of **left recurrent laryngeal nerve injury**. This occurs as a result of the location of the left main pulmonary artery in relation to the aortic arch and recurrent laryngeal nerve, with dissection in this region resulting in direct nerve trauma. **Atrial fibrillation** occurs in 20 % of patients following pneumonectomy. The incidence of atrial (and ventricular) arrhythmias has been significantly reduced by the use of thoracic epidural analgesia. **Pneumonia** following pneumonectomy is a serious complication and can result in **respiratory failure** and death. The incidence of this complication, too, has been reduced by thoracic epidural analgesia. **Empyema** and **abscess formation** are serious complications. Many patients will require a surgical drainage procedure; with the consequential debility, this entails including prolonged hospital stay and other sequelae. Inadvertent **injury to the lung** is also possible especially in the presence of dense pleural adhesions, and occasionally **pneumothorax** or **persistent air leak** may result. Complications specific to the underlying problem and reason for the lung resection may occur. **Basal atelectasis** and sometimes secondary **lung infection** are not uncommon and may affect either lung. **Chylothorax** and **bronchopleural fistula** formation are chronic debilitating problems that delay recovery significantly. **Multisystem organ failure** is extremely serious, the incidence being most related to the underlying lung pathology and other comorbidities, and is associated with mortality.

**Consent and Risk Reduction**

**Main Points to Explain**

- Discomfort
- Bruising and bleeding
- Infection
- Pneumothorax (rare)
- Cardiac arrhythmias (usually minor)
- Failure of insertion
- Catheter displacement/later failure
- Further surgery

# Patent Ductus Arteriosus Ligation

## Description

General anesthesia is used. Patent ductus arteriosus ligation is most commonly undertaken in the neonatal and pediatric age groups. Rarely a late presentation in adulthood is seen. It is described together for all age groups. The aim is to close the patent ductus arteriosus that transmits blood between the aortic arch and the pulmonary trunk. Many small PDAs are closed using radiologically placed intravascular devices, but larger shunts often require surgical closure. The approach is typically via left thoracotomy (neonate), left posterolateral (adults) thoracotomy, or occasionally a median sternotomy; however, thoracoscopic approaches are increasingly being used. Extracorporeal cardiac bypass circuits are seldom required but may be used in older adult patients or with concomitant procedures. Radiological endovascular methods are increasingly being used to close the patent ductus arteriosus.

## *Anatomical Points*

The ductus arteriosus is essential for the conduction of blood from the right heart and pulmonary circulation to the aorta and systemic circulation in utero before birth. At birth, with expansion of the lungs, the pulmonary resistance drops and the blood enters the lungs, with consequent dramatic reduction of the flow via the ductus arteriosus, which contracts closed and then involutes over time to form the ligamentum arteriosum. If closure fails the ductus may remain patent causing a left to right shunt of oxygenated blood from arterial to venous circulations. It is at least twice as common in females as males and also in preterm infants.

## *Perspective*

See Table 5.6. The risk of complications after ductus ligation is related to the size of the preoperative shunt, the age of the patient, and presence of comorbidities. In the neonatal and pediatric patients, the most common problems are similar to those in pediatric thoracic surgery. Major bleeding is usually catastrophic and requires significant transfusion. Infection and recurrent laryngeal nerve injury are also prevalent. Other complications include discomfort, chronic pain, and rarely recurrent pneumothorax, pyothorax, and chylothorax. Neonates are at higher risk of complications associated with prematurity and represent difficulties with transfer to theater, anesthesia, and perioperative care that are unique to this group. Risk is especially high for the premature, extremely low-birth-weight infants and for those with coexisting anomalies. PDA ligation is predominantly to prevent chronic right heart overload and pulmonary hypertension, and these are maximized depending on shunt size and comorbidities. Complications from L–R shunt and from hemodynamic changes after (e.g., NEC, renal dysfunction) are often reduced in the absence (of a shunt, yet may complicate the perioperative management.)

In adult patients the most common problems are similar to those with major thoracic surgery.

Occasionally, cardiopulmonary bypass may be required. Complications include cardiac arrhythmias and chest infection. Bleeding is often catastrophic. Other complications include discomfort, chronic pain, recurrent pneumothorax, pyothorax,

**Table 5.6** Patent ductus arteriosus ligation estimated frequency of complications, risks, and consequences

| Complications, risks, and consequences | Estimated frequency |
|---|---|
| ***Most significant/serious complications*** | |
| Infection | |
|    Subcutaneous/wound | 1–5 % |
|    Intrathoracic (pneumonia, pleural) | 1–5 % |
|    Systemic | 0.1–1 % |
|    Mediastinitis | <0.1 % |
|    Pulmonary empyema or abscess | <0.1 % |
|    Endocarditis (if remains patent) | 1–5 % |
| Pneumothorax | 1–5 % |
| Hemolysis (if remains patent) | 1–5 % |
| Recurrent laryngeal nerve injury | 1–5 % |
| ***Rare significant/serious problems*** | |
| Bleeding/hematoma formation | |
|    Wound | 0.1–1 % |
|    Hemothorax | 0.1–1 % |
|    Pulmonary contusion | 0.1–1 % |
| Surgical emphysema | 0.1–1 % |
| Cardiac arrhythmias | 0.1–1 % |
| Pericardial effusion | 0.1–1 % |
| Esophageal injury[a] | 0.1–1 % |
| Myocardial injury, cardiac failure, MI (hypotension) | 0.1–1 % |
| Pulmonary injury (direct or indirect) | 0.1–1 % |
| Abdominal organ injury[a] | 0.1–1 % |
| Venous thrombosis | 0.1–1 % |
| Further surgery[a] | 0.1–1 % |
| Thoracic duct injury (chylous leak, fistula)[a] | <0.1 % |
| Diaphragmatic injury paresis | <0.1 % |
| Multisystem failure (renal, pulmonary, cardiac failure)[a] | 0.1–1 % |
| Mortality (in term, otherwise normal neonates)[a] | 0.1–1 % |
| Mortality (in premature, low birth weight, and/or with congenital anomalies)[a] | 1–5 % |
| Mortality <u>without</u> surgery[a] | 1–5 % |
| ***Less serious complications*** | |
| Pain/tenderness [rib pain, wound pain] | |
|    Acute (<4weeks) | >80 % |
|    Chronic (>12weeks) | 1–5 % |
| Wound scarring | 5–20 % |
| Deformity of rib/chest or skin (poor cosmesis) | 1–5 % |
| Pleural drain tube(s)[a] | 1–5 % |

[a]Dependent on underlying pathology, comorbidities, severity of anomalies, location of disease, and/or surgical preference

chylothorax, and pulmonary embolism. Ligation of small PDA is typically associated with relatively few major complications. Overall, the most common problems associated with PDA surgery are **bleeding, recurrent laryngeal nerve injury, cardiac arrhythmias,** and **chest infection**. **Stroke** is very rare but is a serious problem when it occurs. **Keloid scar** formation may be severe, irritating, and unsightly.

## Major Complications

**Bleeding**, although rare, can be catastrophic. **Infection** and **recurrent laryngeal injury** are also relatively common. Other complications specific to surgery are rare and usually reflect risks of prematurity. **Stroke, pneumonia, lung abscess, and severe arrhythmias** represent serious complications, which are fortunately rare, although more common in adults and those with preexisting cardiac problems, but can be fatal. **Reoperation** may rarely be required. **Multisystem organ failure** prolongs ICU care and can be associated with cardiac failure, often related to underlying morbidity. In pediatric patients this is associated with extreme prematurity and anomalies; in adults it is associated with preexisting preoperative conditions, such as diabetes, renal failure, cardiac failure, aortic disease, lung disease, advanced age, and recent smoking history (often with or without operation). Mortality risk is increased by existing congenital anomalies (often with or without operation).

---

**Consent and Risk Reduction**

**Main Points to Explain**

- GA risk
- Wound infection
- Bleeding
- Cardiac arrhythmias
- Stroke
- Respiratory infection
- Chest wall pain
- Respiratory or renal failure
- Nerve injury and voice changes
- Further surgery, including reoperation
- Death

---

# Chest Wall Deformities (Pectus Excavatum)

## Description

General anesthesia is used. Pectus excavatum is a common congenital anomaly, occurring in over 1:500 births, resulting in depression of the anterior chest. It may produce physical symptoms but is often a significant psychological and cosmetic problem. A variety of methods are used for correction, often dependent on the type of deformity. The two principal techniques are (i) limited dissection and the use of a plastic or metal bar or plate to elevate the sternum (Nuss procedure) and (ii) resection of the attachments to the depressed sternum and elevation (Ravitch/Haller procedures). The first being more popular, less invasive, and associated with less complications than the latter ones, which essentially are "thoracotomies." Reoperation for progressive deformities as chest wall growth occurs may be required.

## Anatomical Points

The chest wall can be affected by a variety of deformities including pectus excavatum, pigeon chest (prominence or protrusion of the sternum), asymmetry of the chest, and various shapes of the rib cage and costal margin. Pectus excavatum is the most common of the true deformities, and the degree of depression of the sternum can vary considerably, even to the extent of compression or displacement of the intrathoracic organs.

The type and extent of abnormality can affect the ease, complications, and results of surgery.

## Perspective

See Table 5.7. The range and severity of complications from surgery for pectus excavatum, or other chest wall deformities, is heavily dependent on the type and extent of deformity present, the operation performed, and existing comorbidities. Injury to the pericardium, pleura, diaphragm, lung, or abdominal organs is possible, and complications may arise accordingly. Fortunately, this is rare.

## Major Complications

The major complication directly related to the thoracoplasty approach is **bleeding**, either from the chest wall musculature or the intercostal vessels. **Intercostal neuralgia**, secondary to intercostal nerve injury and/or scarring, can occur and may be permanent in some cases. **Costochondritis** can occur secondary to trauma at the costochondral joints. **Osteomyelitis** is very rare. Inadvertent **injury to the lung** is also possible especially in the presence of dense pleural adhesions, and occasionally **pneumothorax** or **persistent air leak** may result. **Pleuritis, basal atelectasis,** and sometimes secondary **lung infection** are not uncommon and may affect either lung. **Empyema** and **abscess formation** are very rare but are severe if they occur leading to prolonged hospital stay and other sequelae. **Cardiac arrhythmias** are not uncommon, and **pericarditis** is reported. **Multisystem organ failure** is extremely serious but rare, the incidence being most related to any underlying lung pathology, aspiration, and other comorbidities.

**Table 5.7** Chest wall deformities (including pectus excavatum) estimated frequency of complications, risks, and consequences

| Complications, risks, and consequences | Estimated frequency |
|---|---|
| ***Most significant/serious complications*** | |
| Infection | |
|    Subcutaneous/wound | 1–5 % |
|    Intrathoracic (pneumonia, pleural) | 1–5 % |
|    Mediastinitis | 0.1–1 % |
|    Systemic | 0.1–1 % |
| Pneumothorax | 1–5 % |
| Scoliosis[a] | 1–5 % |
| Failure of correction of deformity[a] | 1–5 % |
| Bar movement[a] | 5–20 % |
| Further surgery[a] | 20–50 % |
| ***Rare significant/serious problems*** | |
| Pulmonary empyema | 0.1–1 % |
| Pulmonary abscess | 0.1–1 % |
| Bleeding | 0.1–1 % |
| Hematoma formation | |
|    Wound | 0.1–1 % |
|    Hemothorax | 0.1–1 % |
|    Pulmonary contusion | 0.1–1 % |
| Surgical emphysema | 0.1–1 % |
| Persistent air leak | 0.1–1 % |
| Bronchopleural fistula | 0.1–1 % |
| Arrhythmias | 0.1–1 % |
| Pericardial effusion | 0.1–1 % |
| Myocardial injury, cardiac failure, MI (hypotension) | 0.1–1 % |
| Pulmonary injury (direct or indirect) | 0.1–1 % |
| Abdominal organ injury[a] | 0.1–1 % |
| Venous thrombosis | 0.1–1 % |
| Osteomyelitis of ribs[a] | 0.1–1 % |
| Sternal wire protrusion/erosion/pain (median sternotomy if used)[a] | 0.1–1 % |
| Diaphragmatic injury paresis | <0.1 % |
| Multisystem failure (renal, pulmonary, cardiac failure)[a] | <0.1 % |
| Diaphragmatic hernia[a] | <0.1 % |
| Mortality[a] | <0.1 % |
| ***Less serious complications*** | |
| Pain/tenderness [rib pain, wound pain] | |
|    Acute (<4weeks) | >80 % |
|    Chronic (>12weeks) | 1–5 % |
| Wound scarring | 5–20 % |
| Deformity of rib/chest or skin (poor cosmesis) | 1–5 % |
| Pleural drain tube(s)[a] | 1–5 % |

[a]Dependent on underlying pathology, location of disease, and/or surgical preference

**Consent and Risk Reduction**

**Main Points to Explain**

- GA risk
- Chest wall pain
- Respiratory infection
- Wound infection
- Bleeding
- Cardiac arrhythmias
- Further surgery, including reoperation
- Death*

*Dependent on underlying pathology, location of disease, and/or surgical
preference**

## Surgery for Esophageal Atresia

### Overview

Left untreated, esophageal atresia (OA) is a lethal congenital abnormality. Therefore,
any discussion of the risks and complications needs to take this inescapable fact into
account at the outset. It should also be *noted that operative risks are not fixed enti-
ties* nor completely the same among different institutions or patient groups. OA is
commonly associated with a tracheoesophageal fistula (TOF) from the lower atretic
esophageal pouch, up into the posterior aspect of the trachea above, or at the carina.
Esophageal atresia (OA) with or without TOF may be an isolated anomaly or occur
in conjunction with any number of a recognized spectrum of major malformations,
e.g., Vertebral anomalies, Anal atresia, Cardiac defects, Tracheoesophageal fistula
and/or Esophageal atresia, Renal anomalies and Limb defects (VACTERL) malformations. The appropriate time for surgical intervention will depend on the presence
of coexisting VACTERL anomalies, prematurity, and lung disease. Complications
are immediate, intermediate term, and long term depending on the anomaly and the
surgery required, and these are explained further.

The most common form of tracheoesophageal fistula (TOF) is blind termination of the upper esophagus and a fistula from the lower trachea to the distal
esophagus. A patent esophagus and TOF may also occur. Complete esophageal
atresia without a TOF can occur. The procedure required is dependent on the site
and type of deformity present. A patent esophagus and TOF may require minimal
mobilization and surgery. However, the deformity ranges from minimal to complete agenesis of the esophagus with a long gap, requiring extensive mobilization
and complex surgery, increasing risks of major complications. Surgery may

demand closure of the TOF alone, repeated dilatation and staged approximation of the blind esophageal ends, or esophageal replacement by gastric tube reconstruction or colonic interposition. Additional malformations (e.g., duodenal atresia or anorectal malformations) should be sought and corrected, as the reported incidence is 1–10 % and may precipitate anastomotic leakage. Established pulmonary infection again increases risks. Some 5 % of patients have chromosomal anomalies, and this may also elevate risk.

## Description

General anesthesia and intensive care support are required. A thoracotomy approach is used. The aim of surgery, which is life saving, is ligation/division of the TOF, followed by esophageal anastomosis if possible. When the gap between upper and lower esophageal pouches is too great to enable safe anastomosis, the surgeon proceeds to creation of a feeding gastrostomy. Immediate threats to life are usually rare; however, rapidly evolving respiratory distress from airway soiling by gastric contents or sudden collapse secondary to gastric perforation due to gaseous distension will mandate immediate surgical intervention in the first hours of life. Established aspiration pneumonitis or coexisting congenital heart disease will usually preclude a safe attempt to ligate the TOF. About 1 in 20 such infants are never weaned from assisted ventilation and succumb.

## Anatomical Points

Anatomical variations largely determine the surgical correction necessary, ranging from a small fistula between the esophagus and trachea with a relatively normal esophagus to complete agenesis of the esophagus with a massive distal tracheal fistula. Associated aortic arch anomalies may render surgery more difficult, including duplex aortic arches. The location of the recurrent laryngeal nerves may be altered by vascular anomalies. Chest wall deformities such as pectus excavatum and scoliosis may alter the ease of approach and therefore the complications. Fusion of some of the lung fissures may occur making the dissection more difficult. The most common *pulmonary vascular* variation involves the pulmonary venous supply. In 10 % of patients the right middle lobe pulmonary vein drains directly into the inferior pulmonary vein rather than the superior pulmonary vein. In 2–5 % of patients, there may be a single pulmonary vein receiving tributaries from all lobes. The lobar pulmonary arterial and venous supply is very variable, thus necessitating careful dissection and identification of individual lobar and segmental vessels prior to ligation and transection. Anatomical variation of the *bronchial tree* is much less common than that of vascular supply. The intra- and extra-pericardial courses of the pulmonary vessels are quite variable and may necessitate the opening of the pericardium for full assessment.

**Table 5.8** Tracheoesophageal fistula and esophageal atresia estimated frequency of complications, risks, and consequences

| Complications, risks, and consequences | Estimated frequency |
|---|---|
| *Most significant/serious complications* | |
| Immediate threats to life | |
|   Aspiration pneumonitis | 5–20 % |
|   Congenital heart disease[a] | 5–20 % |
|   Cardiac arrhythmias[a] | 5–20 % |
|   Pneumonia[a] | 20–50 % |
|   Multisystem organ failure[a] | 20–50 % |
|   Death (with surgery)[a] | 20–50 % |
|   Death (<u>without</u> surgery)[a] | 100 % |
| Early postoperative | |
|   Anastomotic leak[a] | 20–50 % |
|   *Radiologically evident* | 30 % |
|   *Clinically significant* | 10 % |
|   Anastomotic disruption[a] (2 %) | 1–5 % |
|   Tracheal repair breakdown (1 %) | 1–5 % |
| Complications in infancy | |
|   Anastomotic stenosis[a] (50 %) | 20–50 % |
|   Anastomotic stricture[a] (20 %) | 5–20 % |
|   GOReflux/esophagitis | >80 % |
|   Gastric fundoplication (33 %) | 20–50 % |
| Complications in childhood | |
|   Esophageal dysmotility (25 %) | 20–50 % |
|   Food bolus obstruction | 5–20 % |
|   GOReflux/esophagitis | >80 % |
| Complications in adulthood | |
|   Esophageal malignancy[a] | 5–20 % |
| *Less serious complications* | |
| Pain/tenderness [rib pain, wound pain] | |
|   Acute (<4weeks) | 50–80 % |
|   Chronic (>12weeks) | 0.1–1 % |
| Surgical emphysema | 0.1–1 % |
| Wound scarring | 5–20 % |
| Deformity of rib/chest or skin (poor cosmesis) | 1–5 % |
| Pleural drain tube(s)[a] | 50–80 % |

[a]Dependent on underlying pathology, severity, location of disease, and/or surgical preference
(%) rates in brackets are more concise individualized values, possibly closer to the reported figures

## Perspective

See Table 5.8. Given the certainty of death without surgery, the relative risks of surgery tend to be more accepted than for many elective or semi-elective procedures. However, every attempt is made to appropriately select the correct patients and procedures to improve surgical outcomes. Unless the infant has lethal CHD or lethal complications of prematurity, the surgical attempt to close the TOF will usually be undertaken. In Australia and some other countries, the coexistence of some chromosomal abnormalities (e.g., Trisomy 21) is not usually regarded as a contraindication for surgical correction; however, this may vary in other regions. The malformation and additional anomalies largely determine the complexity of corrective surgery and risk of complications. Complications are common in the immediate postoperative period but also extend into later life, with some not being apparent until adulthood. Clearly, anastomotic leakage is a significant problem if it is large or causes infection, but some small leaks seal spontaneously. Subsequent surgery for diversion or repair may be required, including re-thoracotomy. Significant risks are present from established infection when this occurs. In one recent study, the mortality and morbidity rates were 24 % and 67 %, respectively, and the most common cause of death was sepsis. The weight of approximately 40 % patients was below the 10th percentile at 2 years of age. Pleural space infection (empyema) is more common following leakage. Bronchopleural or esophagocutaneous fistulae represent significant problems. Intercostal neuralgia and numbness/paresthesia of the chest wall can occur. Social problems from prolonged or repeated hospitalizations are also not uncommon.

## Major Complications

### Early Postoperative Complications

**Anastomotic leakage from the esophagus** is seen to some degree in about 30 % of cases. Commonly, this is subclinical, only apparent on contrast swallow performed a few days postsurgery. Subclinical leaks are contained near the anastomosis and usually heal spontaneously over days. However, about 10 % esophageal anastomoses are complicated by a clinically significant leak. This will necessitate control by well-placed chest drains, sometimes requiring an early **second thoracotomy** to lavage the mediastinum and place the drains appropriately. Complete disruption of the anastomosis is seen in about 2 % of cases, usually in the setting of the original attempt involving esophageal ends which are widely separated, termed "long-gap" OA. **Death** is inevitable without immediate cervical esophagostomy or second thoracotomy and reanastomosis. **Breakdown of the tracheal repair** is very rare (1 %) and seen only in the immediate postoperative period. **Atrial fibrillation** and ventricular arrhythmias occur in 5–20 % of patients.

### Later Complications

Complications in Infancy: **Anastomotic stenosis** necessitating at least one subsequent balloon or bougie **esophageal dilatation** is common before 3 months of age (50 %). Development of a mature **esophageal stricture**, at times exacerbated by **esophagitis** secondary to reflux, occurs in approximately 20 % of cases, requiring repeated dilatation for up to the first year of life. **Gastroesophageal reflux** is virtually universal, mandating initial **anti-reflux medical therapy** in infancy, with around a third of all OA children subsequently having a **gastric fundoplication**.

Complications in Childhood: Gastroesophageal reflux and reflux esophagitis are previously discussed. **Esophageal dysmotility** is universal to some degree and

**Table 5.9** Some more individualized concise frequencies of esophageal atresia and surgery according to age ranges

|                            | Complication                   | Incidence   |
| -------------------------- | ------------------------------ | ----------- |
| Immediate threats to life  | Aspiration pneumonitis         | Individual  |
|                            | Congenital heart disease       | Individual  |
|                            | Other anomalies                | Individual  |
|                            | Death                          | Individual  |
| Early postoperative        | Anastomotic leak               |             |
|                            | *Radiologically evident*       | 30 %        |
|                            | *Clinically significant*       | 10 %        |
|                            | Anastomotic disruption         | 2 %         |
|                            | Tracheal repair breakdown      | 1 %         |
| Complications in infancy   | Anastomotic stenosis           | 50 %        |
|                            | Anastomotic stricture          | 20 %        |
|                            | GOReflux/esophagitis           | >95 %       |
|                            | Gastric fundoplication         | 33 %        |
| Complications in childhood | Esophageal dysmotility         | 25 %        |
|                            | Food bolus obstruction         | 5–20 %      |
|                            | GOReflux/esophagitis           | >80 %       |
| Complications in adulthood | Esophageal malignancy          | Individual  |

clinically significant in approximately 25 %. These children often need to drink a mouthful following a bread or sausage meat bolus. When this behavior is momentarily forgotten, some foods may fail to pass through the lower esophagus, causing **bolus obstruction** sometimes needing **endoscopic removal**. Thus, 1–2 re-presentations each for food bolus obstruction during toddlerhood are common in these patients.

Complications in Adulthood: The first surviving infant was in 1945 in the USA, so complete lifetime collective data are not yet available. Worryingly, however, adults with OA are presenting with **esophageal malignancy** at an earlier age than is seen in the general population, with several deaths reported for previously well people in their 5th decade. The etiology is uncertain although undiagnosed reflux/esophagitis/dysplasia is currently considered the most likely cause.

**Pulmonary edema** can result in subsequent cardiac compromise, being difficult to treat, with a high mortality. Another significant complication is **(left) recurrent laryngeal nerve injury**. This occurs as a result of the location of the left main pulmonary artery in relation to the aortic arch and recurrent laryngeal nerve, where dissection in this region can result in direct nerve trauma. **Pneumonia** is a serious complication and can result in **respiratory failure** and **death**. **Empyema** and **abscess formation** are serious complications, often requiring a surgical drainage procedure, with prolonged hospital stay and other sequelae. Inadvertent **injury to the lung** may occur especially in the presence of dense pleural adhesions, and occasionally **pneumothorax** or **persistent air leak** may result. **Chylothorax** and **bronchopleural fistula** formation are chronic debilitating problems that delay recovery significantly. **Multisystem organ failure** is extremely serious, the incidence being most related to the underlying pathology and other comorbidities, and is associated with high mortality. **Mortality** is greater for infants with long separation atresia and in very preterm/low birth weight (<1,500 g), especially in association with serious chromosomal anomalies. See Table 5.9.

**Consent and Risk Reduction**

**Main Points to Explain**

- Risks without surgery
- GA risk
- Bleeding/hematoma
- Infection (local/systemic)*
- Pneumonia
- Anastomotic leak
- Stricture
- Cardiac arrhythmias
- Multisystem organ failure
- Death (with surgery)
- Death (without surgery)
- Possible further surgery*

***Dependent on pathology, comorbidities, and surgery performed**


# Further Reading, References, and Resources

## *Bronchoscopy and/or Extraction of Respiratory Foreign Bodies*

Ashcraft KW, Holcomb GW, Murphy JP, editors. Ashcraft's pediatric surgery. 5th ed. Philadelphia: Saunders/Elsevier; 2009. ISBN: 9781416061274.

Baue AE, Geha AS, Hammond GL, et al. Glen's thoracic & cardiovascular surgery. 6th ed. Stamford: Appleton & Lange; 1996.

Caty MG. Complications in pediatric surgery. New York: Informa Healthcare; 2008. ISBN 9780824728366.

Hutson JM, O'Brien M, Woodward AA, Beasley SW. Jones' clinical paediatric surgery: diagnosis & management. 6th ed. Melbourne: Wiley-Blackwell; 2008. ISBN: 978–1405162678.

Sabiston DC, Spencer FC. Surgery of the chest. 5th ed. Philadelphia: WB Saunders; 1990.

Shields TW. General thoracic surgery. 4th ed. Baltimore: Williams & Wilkins; 1994.

Spitz L, Coran AG, editors. Operative pediatric surgery. 6th ed. London: Hodder-Arnold; 2006.

## *Diagnostic Thoracoscopy*

Ashcraft KW, Holcomb GW, Murphy JP, editors. Ashcraft's pediatric surgery. 5th ed. Philadelphia: Saunders/Elsevier; 2009. ISBN: 9781416061274.

Baue AE, Geha AS, Hammond GL, et al. Glen's thoracic & cardiovascular surgery. 6th ed. Stamford: Appleton & Lange; 1996.

Caty MG. Complications in pediatric surgery. New York: Informa Healthcare; 2008. ISBN 9780824728366.

Hutson JM, O'Brien M, Woodward AA, Beasley SW. Jones' clinical paediatric surgery: diagnosis & management. 6th ed. Melbourne: Wiley-Blackwell; 2008. ISBN: 978–1405162678.

Sabiston DC, Spencer FC. Surgery of the chest. 5th ed. Philadelphia: WB Saunders; 1990.

Shields TW. General thoracic surgery. 4th ed. Baltimore: Williams & Wilkins; 1994.
Spitz L, Coran AG, editors. Operative pediatric surgery. 6th ed. London: Hodder-Arnold; 2006.

## Thoracotomy

Ashcraft KW, Holcomb GW, Murphy JP, editors. Ashcraft's pediatric surgery. 5th ed. Philadelphia: Saunders/Elsevier; 2009. ISBN: 9781416061274.
Baue AE, Geha AS, Hammond GL, et al. Glen's thoracic & cardiovascular surgery. 6th ed. Stamford: Appleton & Lange; 1996.
Caty MG. Complications in pediatric surgery. New York: Informa Healthcare; 2008. ISBN 9780824728366.
Hutson JM, O'Brien M, Woodward AA, Beasley SW. Jones' clinical paediatric surgery: diagnosis & management. 6th ed. Melbourne: Wiley-Blackwell; 2008. ISBN: 978–1405162678.
Sabiston DC, Spencer FC. Surgery of the chest. 5th ed. Philadelphia: WB Saunders; 1990
Shields TW. General thoracic surgery. 4th ed. Baltimore: Williams & Wilkins; 1994.
Spitz L, Coran AG, editors. Operative pediatric surgery. 6th ed. London: Hodder-Arnold; 2006.

## Partial Lung Resection

Ashcraft KW, Holcomb GW, Murphy JP, editors. Ashcraft's pediatric surgery. 5th ed. Philadelphia: Saunders/Elsevier; 2009. ISBN: 9781416061274.
Baue AE, Geha AS, Hammond GL, et al. Glen's thoracic & cardiovascular surgery. 6th ed. Stamford: Appleton & Lange; 1996.
Caty MG. Complications in pediatric surgery. New York: Informa Healthcare; 2008. ISBN 9780824728366.
Hutson JM, O'Brien M, Woodward AA, Beasley SW. Jones' Clinical paediatric surgery: diagnosis & management. 6th ed. Melbourne: Wiley-Blackwell; 2008. ISBN: 978–1405162678.
Sabiston DC, Spencer FC. Surgery of the chest. 5th ed. Philadelphia: WB Saunders; 1990.
Shields TW. General thoracic surgery. 4th ed. Baltimore: Williams & Wilkins; 1994.
Spitz L, Coran AG, editors. Operative pediatric surgery. 6th ed. London: Hodder-Arnold; 2006.

## Pneumonectomy

Ashcraft KW, Holcomb GW, Murphy JP, editors. Ashcraft's pediatric surgery. 5th ed. Philadelphia: Saunders/Elsevier; 2009. ISBN: 9781416061274.
Baue AE, Geha AS, Hammond GL, et al. Glen's thoracic & cardiovascular surgery. 6th ed. Stamford: Appleton & Lange; 1996.
Caty MG. Complications in pediatric surgery. New York: Informa Healthcare; 2008. ISBN 9780824728366.
Hutson JM, O'Brien M, Woodward AA, Beasley SW. Jones' Clinical paediatric surgery: diagnosis & management. 6th ed. Melbourne: Wiley-Blackwell; 2008. ISBN: 978–1405162678.
Sabiston DC, Spencer FC. Surgery of the chest. 5th ed. Philadelphia: WB Saunders; 1990.
Shields TW. General thoracic surgery. 4th ed. Baltimore: Williams & Wilkins; 1994
Spitz L, Coran AG, editors. Operative pediatric surgery. 6th ed. London: Hodder-Arnold; 2006.

## Patent Ductus Arteriosus Ligation

Alexander F, Chiu L, Kroh M, Hammel J, Moore J. Analysis of outcome in 298 extremely low-birth-weight infants with patent ductus arteriosus. J Pediatr Surg. 2009;44(1):112–7. discussion 117.

Ashcraft KW, Holcomb GW, Murphy JP, editors. Ashcraft's pediatric surgery. 5th ed. Philadelphia: Saunders/Elsevier; 2009. ISBN: 9781416061274.

Aydin H, Ozisik K. Surgical removal of an embolized patent ductus arteriosus coil from pulmonary artery without cardiopulmonary bypass. Interact Cardiovasc Thorac Surg. 2009;8(6):689–90.

Caty MG. Complications in pediatric surgery. New York: Informa Healthcare; 2008. ISBN 9780824728366.

Chen ZY, Wu LM, Luo YK, Lin CG, Peng YF, Zhen XC, Chen LL. Comparison of long-term clinical outcome between transcatheter Amplatzer occlusion and surgical closure of isolated patent ductus arteriosus. Chin Med J (Engl). 2009;122(10):1123–7.

Chiruvolu A, Jaleel MA. Therapeutic management of patent ductus arteriosus. Early Hum Dev. 2009;85(3):151–5.

Clemente CD. Anatomy – a regional atlas of the human body. 4th ed. Baltimore: Williams and Wilkins; 1997.

Dani C, Bertini G, Corsini I, Elia S, Vangi V, Pratesi S, Rubaltelli FF. The fate of ductus arteriosus in infants at 23–27 weeks of gestation: from spontaneous closure to ibuprofen resistance. Acta Paediatr. 2008;97(9):1176–80.

Daniels SR. Could PDA, ligation be a course of bronchopulmonary dysplasia? J Pediatr. 2009;154(6):A2.

Dodge-Khatami A, Tschuppert S, Latal B, Rousson V, Doell C. Late morbidity during childhood and adolescence in previously premature neonates after patent ductus arteriosus closure. Pediatr Cardiol. 2009;30(6):735–40.

Giardini A, Derrick G. The effect of ductal diameter on surgical and medical closure of patent ductus arteriosus in preterm neonates. J Thorac Cardiovasc Surg. 2008;136(1):240; author reply 240.

Hobo K, Hanayama N, Umezu K, Shimada N, Toyama A, Takazawa A. Adult patent ductus arteriosus: successful surgery with mitral valvuloplasty. Asian Cardiovasc Thorac Ann. 2009;17(3):302–3.

Hutson JM, O'Brien M, Woodward AA, Beasley SW. Jones' Clinical paediatric surgery: diagnosis & management. 6th ed. Melbourne: Wiley-Blackwell; 2008. ISBN: 978–1405162678.

Inaba H, Higuchi K, Koseni K, Osawa H, Kinoshita O. Surgical closure of adult patent ductus arteriosus using a pursestring suture. Asian Cardiovasc Thorac Ann. 2008;16(1):59–61.

Jamieson GG. The anatomy of general surgical operations. 2 ed. Edinburgh: Churchill Livingston; 2006.

Lin CC, Hsieh KS, Huang TC, Weng KP. Closure of large patent ductus arteriosus in infants. Am J Cardiol. 2009;103(6):857–61.

Lukish JR. Video-assisted thoracoscopic ligation of a patent ductus arteriosus in a very low-birth-weight infant using a novel retractor. J Pediatr Surg. 2009;44(5):1047–50.

Madan JC, Kendrick D, Hagadorn JI, Frantz 3rd ID, National Institute of Child Health and Human Development Neonatal Research Network. Patent ductus arteriosus therapy: impact on neonatal and 18-month outcome. Pediatrics. 2009;123(2):674–81.

Malviya M, Ohlsson A, Shah S. Surgical versus medical treatment with cyclooxygenase inhibitors for symptomatic patent ductus arteriosus in preterm infants. Cochrane Database Syst Rev. 2008;23(1):CD003951. Review.

Mandhan P, Brown S, Kukkady A, Samarakkody U. Surgical closure of patent ductus arteriosus in preterm low birth weight infants. Congenit Heart Dis. 2009;4(1):34–7.

Prada F, Mortera C, Bartrons J, Rissech M, Jiménez L, Carretero J, Llevadias J, Araica M. Percutaneous treatment of atrial septal defects, muscular ventricular septal defects and patent ductus arteriosus in infants under one year of age. Rev Esp Cardiol. 2009;62(9):1050–4.

Sivakumar K, Francis E, Krishnan P. Safety and feasibility of transcatheter closure of large patent ductus arteriosus measuring >or=4 mm in patients weighing <or=6 kg. J Interv Cardiol. 2008;21(2):196–203.

Spanos WC, Brookes JT, Smith MC, Burkhart HM, Bell EF, Smith RJ. Unilateral vocal fold paralysis in premature infants after ligation of patent ductus arteriosus: vascular clip versus suture ligature. Ann Otol Rhinol Laryngol. 2009;118(10):750–3.

Spitz L, Coran AG, editors. Operative pediatric surgery. 6th ed. London: Hodder-Arnold; 2006.

Tanoue Y, Masuda M, Eto M, Tominaga R. Patent ductus arteriosus with hemiazygos communication to left superior vena cava. Ann Thorac Cardiovasc Surg. 2008;14(4):256–7.

Vanderhaegen J, De Smet D, Meyns B, Van De Velde M, Van Huffel S, Naulaers G. Surgical closure of the patent ductus arteriosus and its effect on the cerebral tissue oxygenation. Acta Paediatr. 2008;97(12):1640–4.

Vida VL, Lago P, Salvatori S, Boccuzzo G, Padalino MA, Milanesi O, Speggiorin S, Stellin G. Is there an optimal timing for surgical ligation of patent ductus arteriosus in preterm infants? Ann Thorac Surg. 2009;87(5):1509–15. discussion 1515–6.

# Chest Wall Deformities (Including Pectus Excavatum)

Ashcraft KW, Holcomb GW, Murphy JP, editors. Ashcraft's pediatric surgery. 5th ed. Philadelphia: Saunders/Elsevier; 2009. ISBN: 9781416061274.

Baue AE, Geha AS, Hammond GL, et al. Glen's thoracic & cardiovascular surgery. 6th ed. Stamford: Appleton & Lange; 1996.

Caty MG. Complications in pediatric surgery. New York: Informa Healthcare; 2008. ISBN 9780824728366.

Hutson JM, O'Brien M, Woodward AA, Beasley SW. Jones' clinical paediatric surgery: diagnosis & management. 6th ed. Melbourne: Wiley-Blackwell; 2008. ISBN: 978–1405162678.

Sabiston DC, Spencer FC. Surgery of the chest. 5th ed. Philadelphia: WB Saunders; 1990.

Shields TW. General thoracic surgery. 4th ed. Baltimore: Williams & Wilkins; 1994.

Spitz L, Coran AG, editors. Operative pediatric surgery. 6th ed. London; Hodder-Arnold; 2006.

# Tracheoesophageal Fistula and Esophageal Atresia

Ashcraft KW, Holcomb GW, Murphy JP. Pediatric surgery. 4th ed. Philadelphia: Elsevier/Saunders; 2005. ISBN: 978–0721602226.

Caty MG. Complications in paediatric surgery. London: Informa Healthcare; 2009. ISBN: 978–0824728366.

de Jong EM, Felix JF, de Klein A, Tibboel D. Etiology of Esophageal Atresia and Tracheoesophageal Fistula: "Mind the Gap". Curr Gastroenterol Rep. 2010;12(3):215–22.

Dutta HK, Harsh S. Embryogenesis of esophageal atresia: is localized vascular accident a factor? J Indian Assoc Pediatr Surg. 2009;14(2):73–5.

Gallo G, Zwaveling S, Groen H, Van der Zee D, Hulscher J. Long-gap esophageal atresia: a metaanalysis of jejunal interposition, colon interposition, and gastric pull-up. Eur J Pediatr Surg. 2012;22(6):420–5.

Goyal A, Jones MO, Couriel JM, Losty PD. Oesophageal atresia and tracheoesophageal fistula. Arch Dis Child Fetal Neonatal Ed. 2006;91(5):F381–4.

Holcomb III GW, Murphy JP. Ashcraft's pediatric surgery. 5th ed. Philadelphia: Elsevier/Saunders; 2010. ISBN 13: 978–1416061274.

Holcomb III GW, Rothenberg SS, Bax KMA, Martinez-Ferro M, Albanese CT, Ostlie DJ, van Der Zee DC, Yeung CK. Thoracoscopic repair of esophageal atresia and tracheoesophageal fistula: a multi-institutional analysis. Ann Surg. 2005;242(3):422–30.

http://en.wikipedia.org/wiki/Tracheoesophageal_fistula. Accessed June 2011.

Hunter CJ, Petrosyan M, Connelly ME, Ford HR, Nguyen NX. Repair of long-gap esophageal atresia: gastric conduits may improve outcome – a 20-year single center experience. Pediatr Surg Int. 2009;25(12):1087–91.

Jamieson GG, editor. The anatomy of general surgical operations. Edinburgh: Churchill-Livingstone/Elsevier; 2006.

Kovesi T, Rubin S. Long-term complications of congenital esophageal atresia and/or tracheoesophageal fistula. Chest. 2004;126(3):915–25.

Puri P, Holwarth M. Paediatric surgery: diagnosis and treatment. Heidelberg: Springer-Verlag; 2009. ISBN 978-3-540-69559-2.

Raj Bhurtel D, Losa I. VACTERL (vertebral anomalies, anal atresia or imperforate anus, cardiac anomalies, tracheoesophageal fistula, renal and limb defect) spectrum presenting with portal hypertension: a case report. J Med Case Rep. 2010;4:128.

Saxena P, Tam R. Late manifestation of a large congenital tracheoesophageal fistula in an adult. Tex Heart Inst J. 2006;33(1):60–2.

Seo J, Kim DY, Kim AR, Kim DY, Kim SC, Kim IK, Kim KS, Yoon CH, Pi SY. An 18-year experience of tracheoesophageal fistula and esophageal atresia. Korean J Pediatr. 2010;53(6):705–10.

Shaw Smith C. Oesophageal atresia, tracheoesophageal fistula, and the VACTERL association: review of genetics and epidemiology. J Med Genet. 2006;43(7):545–54.

Shaw-Smith C. Genetic factors in esophageal atresia, tracheo-esophageal fistula and the VACTERL association: roles for FOXF1 and the 16q24.1 FOX transcription factor gene cluster, and review of the literature. Eur J Med Genet. 2010;53(1–3):6–13.

Spitz L. Oesophageal atresia. Orphanet J Rare Dis. 2007; 2:24.

van der Zee DC, Vieirra-Travassos D, de Jong JR, Tytgat SHAJ. A novel technique for risk calculation of anastomotic leakage after thoracoscopic repair of esophageal atresia with distal fistula. World J Surg. 2008;32(7):1396–9.

van der Zee DC, Tytgat SH, Zwaveling S, van Herwaarden MY, Vieira-Travassos D. Learning curve of thoracoscopic repair of esophageal atresia. World J Surg. 2012;36(9):2093–7.

# Chapter 6
# Pediatric Vascular Access Surgery

Anthony L. Sparnon, Christine Russell, and Brendon J. Coventry

## General Perspective and Overview

The relative risks and complications increase proportionately according to the site, size, and type and complexity of the problem being addressed within the chest and in relation to the age of the patient and other comorbidities. This is principally related to the surgical accessibility, ability to correct the problem, functional reserve, technical ease, and the ability to achieve correction of the problem.

The main serious complications are **bleeding and infection,** which can be minimized by the adequate exposure, mobilization, technical care, and avoiding injury and hematoma formation. Infection is the main sequel of tissue injury and hematoma formation and may arise from preexisting infection or be newly acquired. This can lead to **catheter infection** and **systemic sepsis.** Although very rare in children, **multisystem failure** and **death** remain serious potential complications from vascular access surgery and systemic infection.

This chapter therefore attempts to draw together in one place the estimated overall frequencies of the complications associated with vascular access procedures based on information obtained from the literature and experience. Not all patients are at risk of the full range of listed complications. It must be individualized for each

A.L. Sparnon, MBBS, FRACS (✉)
Women's and Children's Hospital, North Adelaide, Australia
e-mail: asparnon@tps.com.au

C. Russell BA, BM, BCh, FRACS
Central and Northern Adelaide Renal and Transplantation Service,
Royal Adelaide Hospital, Adelaide, Australia
e-mail: christine.russell3@health.sa.gov.au

B.J. Coventry, BMBS, PhD, FRACS, FACS, FRSM
Discipline of Surgery, Royal Adelaide Hospital, University of Adelaide,
L5 Eleanor Harrald Building, North Terrace, 5000 Adelaide, SA, Australia
e-mail: brendon.coventry@adelaide.edu.au

B.J. Coventry (ed.), *Pediatric Surgery*, Surgery: Complications, Risks and Consequences,     157
DOI 10.1007/978-1-4471-5439-6_6, © Springer-Verlag London 2014

**Important Note**

It should be emphasized that the risks and frequencies that are given here *represent derived figures*. These *figures are best estimates of relative frequencies across most institutions*, not merely the highest-performing ones, and as such are often representative of a number of studies, which include different patients with differing comorbidities and different surgeons. In addition, the risks of complications in lower- or higher-risk patients may lie outside these estimated ranges, and individual clinical judgment is required as to the expected risks communicated to the patient and staff or for other purposes. The range of risks is also derived from experience and the literature; while risks outside this range may exist, certain risks may be reduced or absent due to variations of procedures or surgical approaches. It is recognized that different patients, practitioners, institutions, regions, and countries may vary in their requirements and recommendations.

patient and their disease process but represents a guide and summary of the attendant risks, complications, and consequences.

With these factors and facts in mind, the information given in this chapter must be appropriately and discernibly interpreted and used.

For complications related to other associated/additional surgery that may arise during vascular access surgery, see the relevant volume and chapter.

# Central Venous Catheter Line Insertion

## Description

General anesthesia is required with an ultrasound or image intensifier available to assist in direct venous access. The aim is to gain access to either the subclavian or internal jugular vein by direct puncture using a percutaneous Seldinger technique (guide wire, dilator, separable sheath, Silastic catheter). Once inserted into the vein, the sheath can be stripped away, leaving the venous catheter. Alternatively, an open approach can be used, although this is more traumatic to the vein and is generally reserved for situations where percutaneous access is difficult or inadvisable. The skin puncture rarely requires closure, and usually a waterproof dressing is all that is needed.

## Anatomical Points

The position of the subclavian and internal jugular veins is relatively constant, although there is some minor variation, due to differences in anatomy between individuals and the hydration status of the patient. Dehydration decreases venous size

**Table 6.1** Central venous line insertion estimated frequency of complications, risks, and consequences

| Complications, risks, and consequences | Estimated frequency |
|---|---|
| *Most significant/serious complications* | |
| Infection (overall) | 5–20 % |
| Wound | 5–20 % |
| Within the catheter | 5–20 % |
| Systemic sepsis | 1–5 % |
| Bleeding/hematoma formation (wound) | 1–5 % |
| Thrombosis – SVC thrombosis/internal jugular/cephalic vein | 5–20 % |
| Migration/displacement of the catheter tube | 1–5 % |
| Catheter failure (late; from whatever cause) | 5–20 % |
| Radiation exposure (for the patient) (low level)[a] | >80 % |
| *Rare significant/serious problems* | |
| Pneumothorax | 0.1–1 % |
| Cardiac arrhythmias (catheter irritation of endocardium) | 0.1–1 % |
| Nerve injury (depending on positioning) | 0.1–1 % |
| Cutaneous nerve, vagus X nerve damage, etc. | |
| Failure to perform catheter insertion (technical problems) | 0.1–1 % |
| Catheter tip embolus | 0.1–1 % |
| Hemothorax | <0.1 % |
| Air embolism | <0.1 % |
| Subclavian vein fistula | <0.1 % |
| Multisystem organ failure[a] | <0.1 % |
| Death[a] | <0.1 % |
| *Less serious complications* | |
| Bruising | 5–20 % |
| Wound dehiscence (open surgery)[a] | 1–5 % |
| Skin/fat necrosis | 0.1–1 % |
| Residual pain/discomfort/neuralgia | 1–5 % |
| Delayed wound healing (incl. ulceration) | 1–5 % |
| Wound scarring (poor cosmesis) | 1–5 % |

[a]Dependent on underlying pathology, anatomy, surgical technique, preferences, and comorbidities

and can make access more difficult. Placing the patient slightly "head-down" is helpful in dilating the venous system of the head and neck facilitating easier entry of the initial needle and reducing risk of air embolism. The pleura lies behind the medial 1/3 of the clavicle on each side and is at risk of puncture and inducing a pneumothorax.

## Perspective

See Table 6.1. The procedure is usually associated with a low complication rate and most are minor, such as bruising, difficulty gaining access to the vein, and minor superficial infection. Major complications are rare, but can occur, such as pneumothorax, which may require further hospitalization or insertion of an underwater-seal chest drain tube. Cardiac arrhythmias and bleeding are risks during insertion. Immediate withdrawal of the catheter wire or tube several centimeters will usually settle the arrhythmia. Catheter thrombosis, cardiac arrhythmias, and migration of the catheter are also potentially serious as the catheter may require removal and later reinsertion. Percutaneous CVC lines invariably fail over time due to infection, mechanical problems, or thrombosis, and regular replacement may avert these issues as clinical complications. Failure to complete the procedure by the percutaneous method will not usually disallow its insertion, since the open approach can then usually be safely used. Bilateral attempts at central line insertion via the subclavian approach at the same operation are not advisable within 24 h, as there is a risk of inducing bilateral pneumothoraces. Use of the internal jugular approach is preferable after a failed subclavian approach.

## Major Complications

The main severe acute complications are **pneumothorax, cardiac arrhythmias, air embolism,** and **hemothorax.** Later, **infection** of the catheter line can lead to **systemic sepsis** and even **multisystem organ failure**, which is the major cause of **mortality**, especially in immunocompromised patients and severely ill patients. **Removal of the central line** invariably follows infection. Air embolism and hemothorax are very rare but can be life threatening. **Catheter blockage or leakage** due to a variety of problems, usually later, may require removal and reinsertion or adjustment. **Catheter thrombosis** and **pulmonary embolism** can occur and may be serious. **Axillary, subclavian, internal jugular, or superior vena cava venous** thrombosis can cause severe swelling of the arm, neck, head, and chest. **Carotid artery puncture** is minimized by the use of ultrasound guidance. **Cardiac arrhythmias** are usually terminated by withdrawal of the guide wire from the heart chamber, usually the atrium affecting the sinoatrial node.

**Consent and Risk Reduction**

**Main Points to Explain**

- Discomfort
- Bruising and bleeding
- Infection
- Pneumothorax (rare)
- Cardiac arrhythmias (usually minor)
- Failure of insertion
- Catheter displacement/later failure
- Further surgery

# Tunneled Internal Jugular Central Venous Catheter Line Insertion

## Description

General anesthesia is used, with an ultrasound and image intensifier present to assist in insertion and checking position. The aim is to insert the catheter into the internal jugular vein percutaneously (or open) and to tunnel this subcutaneously to a convenient site in the anterior axilla, upper chest, or abdomen for exit and access. The line can be inserted percutaneously or via an open approach. If using the percutaneous route, ultrasound guidance may lower the complication rate. The patient should be placed head-down to avoid an air embolus and the head rotated toward the other side to give more access. When using the open approach, a cervical skin crease incision is placed over the carotid pulsation, 1-finger width above the clavicle. The SVC is secured above and below the venotomy site and the largest catheter for the vein size is inserted. A circumferential 6/0 Prolene suture closes the venotomy against the catheter. Some catheters have a small Dacron cuff, which is positioned under the skin, to fixate the catheter.

## Anatomical Points

The position of the subclavian and internal jugular veins is relatively constant; however, there is some relative variation between individuals and the hydration status of the patient. Dehydration decreases venous size and can make access more difficult. The internal jugular vein can overlie or even be medial to the carotid artery in some patients, and ultrasound guidance may be of value. The pleura lies behind the medial 1/3 of the clavicle on each side and is at risk of puncture and inducing a pneumothorax. Great care with the tunneling is required to avoid possible damage to the breast bud in girls as subsequent hypoplasia or problems in growth may develop.

## Perspective

See Table 6.2. The procedure is usually associated with a low complication rate and most are minor, such as bruising, difficulty gaining access to the vein, and minor superficial infection. Life-threatening complications are rare and less common by the open compared with the subclavian route. Major complications are rare, but can occur, such as pneumothorax, which may require further hospitalization or insertion of an underwater-seal chest drain tube. Air embolus is very rare, especially if the "head-down" patient position is used, which is also helpful in dilating the venous system of the head and neck facilitating easier entry of the initial needle. Cardiac

**Table 6.2** Tunneled internal jugular line insertion estimated frequency of complications, risks, and consequences

| Complications, risks, and consequences | Estimated frequency |
|---|---|
| *Most significant/serious complications* | |
| Infection (overall) | 20–50 % |
|   Wound | 1–5 % |
|   Related to the catheter | 5–20 % |
|   Systemic sepsis | 1–5 % |
| Bruising | 20–50 % |
| Extravasation or bleeding/hematoma formation | 1–5 % |
| Thrombosis – SVC thrombosis/internal jugular/cephalic vein | 1–5 % |
| Seroma/lymphocele/lymphatic leak | 1–5 % |
| Failure to perform catheter insertion (technical problems) | 1–5 % |
|   (Depends on number of previous catheterizations in dialysis patients and use of U/S) | |
| Catheter failure (from whatever cause) | 1–5 % |
|   [Misdirection; occlusion; kinking; fracture/breakage; too long/short] | |
| *Rare significant/serious problems* | |
| Pneumothorax (rare with internal jugular cannulation) | 0.1–1 % |
| Cather malposition | 0.1–1 % |
| Cardiac arrhythmias (catheter irritation of endocardium) | 0.1–1 % |
| Migration/displacement of the catheter tube | 0.1–1 % |
| Vessel perforation and hemorrhage | <0.1 % |
| Hemothorax (rare with internal jugular cannulation) | <0.1 % |
| Laryngeal edema | <0.1 % |
| Cardiac perforation and tamponade | <0.1 % |
| Air embolism | <0.1 % |
| Nerve injury (depending on positioning) | <0.1 % |
|   Cutaneous nerve, vagus X nerve damage, etc. | |
| Catheter tip embolus | <0.1 % |
| Breast bud growth problems | <0.1 % |
| Multisystem organ failure[a] | <0.1 % |
| Death[a] | <0.1 % |
| *Less serious complications* | |
| Wound dehiscence | 1–5 % |
| Skin necrosis | 0.1–1 % |
| Residual pain/discomfort/neuralgia | 1–5 % |
| Delayed wound healing (incl. ulceration) | 1–5 % |
| Wound scarring (poor cosmesis) | 1–5 % |
| Failure of breast bud development | <0.1 % |

[a]Dependent on underlying pathology, anatomy, surgical technique, preferences, and comorbidities

arrhythmias and bleeding are risks during insertion. Immediate withdrawal of the catheter wire or tube several centimeters will usually settle the arrhythmia. Catheter thrombosis, cardiac arrhythmias, and migration of the catheter are also potentially serious as the catheter may require removal and later reinsertion. Percutaneous CVC lines invariably fail over time due to infection, mechanical problems, or thrombosis, and regular replacement may avert these issues as clinical complications. Failure to complete the procedure by the percutaneous method will not usually disallow its insertion, since the open approach can usually be then used. Bilateral attempts at central line insertion at the same operation are not advisable within 24 h, as there is a very small, but important, risk of inducing bilateral pneumothoraces. Use of the open internal jugular approach can then be used. Great care with the tunneling is required to avoid possible damage to the breast bud in girls as subsequent hypoplasia or problems in growth may develop. Migration of the catheter is rare as textured cuff is incorporated by the surrounding tissues and usually holds it in place.

## Major Complications

The main severe acute complications are **pneumothorax, cardiac arrhythmias, air embolism,** and **hemothorax.** Later, **infection** of the catheter line can lead to **systemic sepsis** and even **multisystem organ failure**, which is the major cause of **mortality**, especially in immunocompromised patients and severely ill patients. **Removal of the central line** invariably follows infection. Air embolism and hemothorax are very rare but can be life threatening. **Catheter blockage or leakage** due to a variety of problems, usually later, may require removal and reinsertion or adjustment. **Catheter thrombosis** and **pulmonary embolism** can occur and may be serious. **Catheter migration** is rare. Rarely, **breast bud development problems** can occur if the catheter tubing is tunneled too close to the nipple in the female child. **Axillary, subclavian, internal jugular, or superior vena cava venous** thrombosis can cause severe swelling of the arm, neck, head, and chest. **Carotid artery puncture** is minimized by the use of ultrasound guidance. **Cardiac arrhythmias** are usually terminated by withdrawal of the guide wire from the heart chamber, usually the atrium affecting the sinoatrial node.

---

**Consent and Risk Reduction**

**Main Points to Explain**

- Discomfort
- Bruising and bleeding
- Infection
- Pneumothorax (rare)
- Cardiac arrhythmias (usually minor)
- Failure of insertion
- Catheter displacement/later failure
- Further surgery

## Open/Percutaneous Venous Access Devices (Infusion-Port) Insertion

### Description

Under general anesthesia, access to either the subclavian or internal jugular vein is obtained using an open or percutaneous approach. The aim is to gain access to the subclavian or internal jugular vein by direct puncture using a percutaneous Seldinger technique (guide wire, dilator, separable sheath, Silastic catheter). Once inserted into the vein, the sheath can be stripped away to leave the venous catheter. Alternatively, an open approach can be used, although this is more traumatic to the vein. For an open approach, a transverse cervical skin crease incision is placed over the carotid pulsation, at triangle between the sternoclavicular heads of the sternomastoid muscle, 1-finger breadth above the clavicle to allow room for pressure if a vascular problem develops. The SVC is secured above and below the venotomy site and the largest catheter for the vein size is inserted. A circumferential 6/0 Prolene suture closes the venotomy. A separate subcutaneous pocket is made for the port, attached to the Silastic catheter. The catheter is tunneled to reach the vein. The position of the catheter in the superior vena cava can then be checked using image intensification radiology. The skin is then closed to render the whole system subcutaneous.

### Anatomical Points

The position of the subclavian and internal jugular veins is relatively constant; however, there is some relative variation, due to differences in the surrounding bony anatomy between individuals and the hydration status of the patient. Dehydration decreases venous size and can make access more difficult. Placing the patient slightly "head-down" is also helpful in dilating the venous system of the head and neck facilitating easier entry of the initial needle and reducing air embolism. The pleura lies behind the medial 1/3 of the clavicle on each side and is at risk of puncture and inducing a pneumothorax.

### Perspective

See Table 6.3. The procedure is usually associated with a low complication rate and most are minor, such as bruising, difficulty gaining access to the vein, and minor superficial infection. Life-threatening complications are rare and less common than by the subclavian route. Major complications are rare, but can occur, such as pneumothorax, which may require further hospitalization or insertion of an underwater-seal chest drain tube. Air embolus is very rare, especially if the

**Table 6.3** Open/percutaneous venous access devices (including infusion-port) insertion estimated frequency of complications, risks, and consequences

| Complications, risks, and consequences | Estimated frequency |
|---|---|
| ***Most significant/serious complications*** | |
| Infection (overall) | 20–50 % |
|   Wound | 1–5 % |
|   Related to the catheter/port | 5–20 % |
|   Systemic sepsis | 1–5 % |
| Bruising | 20–50 % |
| Extravasation or bleeding/hematoma formation | 1–5 % |
| Thrombosis – SVC thrombosis/internal jugular/cephalic vein | 1–5 % |
| Seroma/lymphocele/lymphatic leak | 1–5 % |
| Failure to perform catheter insertion (technical problems) | 1–5 % |
|   (Depends on number of previous catheterizations in dialysis patients and use of U/S) | |
| Catheter failure (later; from whatever cause) | 1–5 % |
|   [Misdirection; occlusion; kinking; fracture/breakage; too long/short] | |
| Port leakage, rotation, separation from tubing, and skin erosion | 1–5 % |
| ***Rare significant/serious problems*** | |
| Pneumothorax (rare with internal jugular cannulation) | 0.1–1 % |
| Cardiac arrhythmias (catheter irritation of endocardium) | 0.1–1 % |
| Catheter malposition | 0.1–1 % |
| Migration/displacement of the catheter tube | 0.1–1 % |
|   Rare as cuff holds it in place | |
| Hemothorax (rare with internal jugular cannulation) | <0.1 % |
| Nerve injury (depending on positioning) | <0.1 % |
|   Cutaneous nerve, vagus X nerve damage, etc. | |
| Laryngeal edema | <0.1 % |
| Cardiac perforation and tamponade | <0.1 % |
| Catheter tip embolus | <0.1 % |
| Air embolism | <0.1 % |
| Vessel perforation and hemorrhage | <0.1 % |
| Breast bud growth problems | <0.1 % |
| Multisystem organ failure[a] | <0.1 % |
| Death[a] | <0.1 % |
| ***Less serious complications*** | |
| Wound dehiscence | 1–5 % |
| Skin necrosis | 0.1–1 % |
| Residual pain/discomfort/neuralgia | 1–5 % |
| Delayed wound healing (incl. ulceration) | 1–5 % |
| Wound scarring (poor cosmesis) | 1–5 % |
| Failure of breast bud development | <0.1 % |

[a]Dependent on underlying pathology, anatomy, surgical technique, preferences, and comorbidities

"head-down" patient position is used. Catheter thrombosis, cardiac arrhythmias, and migration of the catheter are also potentially serious as the catheter may require removal and later reinsertion. Cardiac arrhythmias and bleeding are risks during insertion. Immediate withdrawal of the catheter wire or tube several centimeters will usually settle the arrhythmia. Catheter thrombosis, cardiac arrhythmias, and migration of the catheter are also potentially serious as the catheter may require removal and later reinsertion. Percutaneous CVC lines and ports invariably fail over time due to infection, mechanical problems, or thrombosis, and regular replacement may avert these issues as clinical complications. Failure to complete the procedure by the percutaneous method will not usually disallow its insertion, since the open approach can usually be then used. Bilateral attempts at central line insertion via the subclavian approach at the same operation are not advisable within 24 h, as there is a risk of inducing bilateral pneumothoraces. Use of the internal jugular approach is preferable after a failed subclavian approach. Pneumothorax risk is about 1 in 200 cannulations via the subcutaneous approach, less with the internal jugular vein route. Problems related to the port include infection, skin necrosis, erosion, rotation, and separation from the tubing. Port rotation can be minimized using careful 3-point fixation of the port and leakage usually prevented by the use of the correct (Huber) needle type. Great care with the tunneling is required to avoid possible damage to the breast bud in girls as subsequent hypoplasia or problems in growth may develop.

## Major Complications

The main severe acute complications with catheter insertion are **pneumothorax, cardiac arrhythmias, air embolism,** and **hemothorax.** Later, **infection** of the catheter line can lead to **systemic sepsis** and even **multisystem organ failure**, which is the major cause of **mortality**, especially in immunocompromised patients and severely ill patients. **Removal of the central line** invariably follows infection. Air embolism and hemothorax are very rare but can be life threatening. **Catheter blockage or leakage** due to a variety of problems, usually later, may require removal and reinsertion or adjustment. **Catheter thrombosis** and **pulmonary embolism** can occur and may be serious. Rarely, **breast bud development problems** can occur if the catheter tubing is tunneled too close to the nipple in the female child. **Axillary, subclavian, internal jugular, or superior vena cava venous** thrombosis can cause severe swelling of the arm, neck, head, and chest. **Carotid artery puncture** is minimized by the use of ultrasound guidance. **Cardiac arrhythmias** are usually terminated by withdrawal of the guide wire from the heart chamber, usually the atrium affecting the sinoatrial node. Problems related to the port include **infection, skin necrosis, erosion**, rotation, and **separation** from the tubing. **Port rotation or leakage/extravasation** requires **further surgery** for adjustment or **port removal**. Rarely, **breast bud development problems** can occur if the catheter tubing is tunneled too close to the nipple in the female child.

**Consent and Risk Reduction**

**Main Points to Explain**

- Discomfort
- Bruising and bleeding
- Infection
- Pneumothorax (rare)
- Cardiac arrhythmias (usually minor)
- Failure of insertion
- Catheter/port displacement/failure
- Further surgery

# Further Reading, References, and Resources

## *Central Venous Line Insertion*

Braner DAV, Susanna Lai, Scott Eman, Ken Tegtmeyer. Central venous catheterization – subclavian vein. N Engl J Med. 2007;357:e26.

Fortune JB, Feustel P. Effect of patient position on size and location of the subclavian vein for percutaneous puncture. Arch Surg. 2003;138:996–1000.

Jamieson GG. The anatomy of general surgical operations. 2nd ed. Edinburgh: Churchill Livingstone; 2006.

Orihashi K, Imai K, Sato K, Hamamoto M, Okada K, Sueda T. Extrathoracic subclavian venipuncture under ultrasound guidance. Circ J. 2005;69:1111–5.

Pirotte T, Veyckemans F. Ultrasound guided subclavian vein cannulation in infants and children: a novel approach. Br J Anaesth. 2007;98:509–14.

## *Tunneled Internal Jugular Line Insertion*

Conlon PJ, Schwab SJ, Nicholson ML, editors. Hemodialysis vascular access: practice and problems. Oxford/New York: Oxford University Press; 2000.

Jamieson GG. The anatomy of general surgical operations. 2nd ed. Edinburgh: Churchill Livingstone; 2006.

Levy J, Morgan J, Brown E, editors. Oxford handbook of dialysis. Haemodialysis. Oxford: Oxford University Press; 2001.

Lin B, Kong C, Tarng D, Huang T, Tang G. Anatomical variation of the internal jugular vein and its impact on temporary haemodialysis vascular access: an ultrasonographic survey in uraemic patients. Nephrol Dial Transplantation. 1998;13:134–8.

## Open/Percutaneous Venous Access Devices
## (Including Infusion-Port) Insertion

Braner DAV, Susanna Lai, Scott Eman, Ken Tegtmeyer. Central venous catheterization – subclavian vein. N Engl J Med. 2007;357:e26.

Conlon PJ, Schwab SJ, Nicholson ML, editors. Hemodialysis vascular access: practice and problems. Oxford/New York: Oxford University Press; 2000.

Fortune JB, Feustel P. Effect of patient position on size and location of the subclavian vein for percutaneous puncture. Arch Surg. 2003;138:996–1000.

Jamieson GG. The anatomy of general surgical operations. 2nd ed. Edinburgh: Churchill Livingstone; 2006.

Lin B, Kong C, Tarng D, Huang T, Tang G. Anatomical variation of the internal jugular vein and its impact on temporary haemodialysis vascular access: an ultrasonographic survey in uraemic patients. Nephrol Dial Transplant. 1998;13:134–8.

Orihashi K, Imai K, Sato K, Hamamoto M, Okada K, Sueda T. Extrathoracic subclavian venipuncture under ultrasound guidance. Circ J. 2005;69:1111–5.

Pirotte T, Veyckemans F. Ultrasound guided subclavian vein cannulation in infants and children: a novel approach. Br J Anaesth. 2007;98:509–14.

# Chapter 7
# Pediatric Urological and Genital Surgery

Hilary Boucaut and Brendon J. Coventry

## General Perspective and Overview

The relative risks and complications increase proportionately according to the site, size, and type and complexity of the problem being addressed within the chest and in relation to the age of the patient and other comorbidities. This is principally related to the surgical accessibility, ability to correct the problem, functional reserve, technical ease, and the ability to achieve correction of the problem.

The main serious complications are **bleeding and infection,** which can be minimized by the adequate exposure, mobilization, technical care, and avoiding injury and hematoma formation. Infection is the main sequel of tissue injury and hematoma formation and may arise from preexisting infection or be newly acquired. This can lead to **urinary infection** and **systemic sepsis**. Although very rare in children, **multisystem failure** and **death** remain serious potential complications from urologic surgery and systemic infection.

This chapter therefore attempts to draw together in one place the estimated overall frequencies of the complications associated with urological procedures, based on information obtained from the literature and experience. Not all patients are at risk of the full range of listed complications. It must be individualized for each patient and their disease process but represents a guide and summary of the attendant risks, complications, and consequences.

With these factors and facts in mind, the information given in this chapter must be appropriately and discernibly interpreted and used.

H. Boucaut, MBBS, FRACS (⊠)
Urology Unit, Women's and Children's Hospital, Adelaide, Australia
e-mail: hboucaut@gmail.com

B.J. Coventry, BMBS, PhD, FRACS, FACS, FRSM
Discipline of Surgery, Royal Adelaide Hospital, University of Adelaide,
L5 Eleanor Harrald Building, North Terrace, 5000 Adelaide, SA, Australia
e-mail: brendon.coventry@adelaide.edu.au

B.J. Coventry (ed.), *Pediatric Surgery*, Surgery: Complications, Risks and Consequences,     169
DOI 10.1007/978-1-4471-5439-6_7, © Springer-Verlag London 2014

**Important Note**
It should be emphasized that the risks and frequencies that are given here *represent derived figures*. These *figures are best estimates of relative frequencies across most institutions*, not merely the highest-performing ones, and as such are often representative of a number of studies, which include different patients with differing comorbidities and different surgeons. In addition, the risks of complications in lower- or higher-risk patients may lie outside these estimated ranges, and individual clinical judgment is required as to the expected risks communicated to the patient and staff or for other purposes. The range of risks is also derived from experience and the literature; while risks outside this range may exist, certain risks may be reduced or absent due to variations of procedures or surgical approaches. It is recognized that different patients, practitioners, institutions, regions, and countries may vary in their requirements and recommendations.

For complications related to other associated/additional surgery that may arise during urological surgery, see the relevant volume and chapter.

## Acknowledgments

The authors would like to acknowledge the contributions and work of several urologists toward aspects of this chapter, Prof Oliver Hakenberg in Germany and Dr John Miller and Prof Villis Marshall in Adelaide who authored the adult chapter and provided information.

## Surgery for Labial Fusion/Adhesions

### *Description*

General anesthesia is usually used for children with this condition. Labial fusion usually occurs after birth, during infancy, as an acquired problem due to inflammation causing adhesions between both labia minora. Labial fusion may be asymptomatic or be associated with vulval irritation, post-micturition dribbling, or urinary tract infections. The aim of treatment is to separate the fused labia to reexpose the vaginal and urethral openings. Primary treatment with topical estrogen cream alone may cause labial separation, but if this fails, manual separation under

**Table 7.1** Surgery for labial fusion/adhesions estimated frequency of complications, risks, and consequences

| Complications, risks, and consequences | Estimated frequency |
|---|---|
| *Most significant/serious complications* | |
| Labial refusion | 5–20 % |
| Further surgery (revision or hematoma drainage) | 1–5 % |
| *Rare significant/serious problems* | |
| Urinary tract infection[a] | 0.1–1 % |
| *Less serious complications* | |
| Labial swelling | 1–5 % |
| Residual pain/discomfort/tenderness | |
| Short term (<2 weeks) | 20–50 % |
| Dysuria | 20–50 % |
| Urinary incontinence/post-micturition dribbling | 0.1–1 % |

[a]Dependent on underlying pathology, anatomy, surgical technique, and preferences

general anesthetic by gently pulling apart of the labia along the line of fusion is all that is usually required.

## Anatomical Points

The fusion is between the free edges of the labia minora extending from the clitoris to the posterior fourchette. The degree of fusion can vary from partial to complete.

## Perspective

See Table 7.1. Complications are generally minor and/or infrequent. Acute dysuria is a typical feature until the skin and mucosa heal. Recurrent fusion is not uncommon, especially in younger girls, and may require repeat separation, until enough labial separation develops as the child grows.

## Major Complications/Consequences

In perspective, there are usually no major complications associated with separation of labial adhesions. **Pain** may rarely be significant requiring regular bathing and pain relief. **Acute dysuria** is a consequence of surgery and is expected, but if prolonged beyond 72 h, it is abnormal. **Urinary tract infection** is very rare and may signify other underlying abnormalities, should it occur. **Bleeding** is rarely severe. **Recurrent labial fusion** is occasionally a frustrating problem that may require further surgical separation.

**Consent and Risk Reduction**

**Main Points to Explain**

- GA risk
- Dysuria
- Pain/discomfort
- Refusion of labia
- Risks without surgery*

# Surgery for Meatal Stenosis

## Description

General anesthesia is used for children. The aim is to dilate the stenosed urethral opening, and a small incision is required. Meatotomy is usually performed by crushing the scar tissue adjacent to the meatus with a clamp and then incising it longitudinally. Sutures are occasionally required for any problematic bleeding. Meatal stenosis is narrowing of the urethral meatus, which can be associated with a previous circumcision as a newborn or infant or can be associated with balanitis xerotica obliterans of the foreskin causing phimosis. The usual presentation is with a fine urinary stream that may spray or be difficult to direct, often with a change in bladder control associated with frequency, urgency, and occasionally incontinence.

## Anatomical Points

The urethral meatus may become stenosed either at the 6 o'clock position alone or at both the 6 and 12 o'clock positions equally.

## Perspective

See Table 7.2. Complications are generally minor and/or infrequent; however, some may be more significant on occasions. These include cosmetic deformity, recurrent meatal stenosis, and bleeding. Brief meatal ulceration is a consequence of surgery and usually heals rapidly. Acute dysuria is a typical feature until the skin and mucosa heal.

## Major Complications/Consequences

In perspective, there are usually no major complications associated with meatotomy. **Pain** may rarely be significant requiring regular bathing and pain relief. **Acute**

**Table 7.2** Surgery for meatal stenosis estimated frequency of complications, risks, and consequences

| Complications, risks, and consequences | Estimated frequency |
|---|---|
| *Most significant/serious complications* | |
| Infection[a] overall | 1–5 % |
|   Urinary | 1–5 % |
| Meatal restenosis | 1–5 % |
| *Rare significant/serious problems* | |
| Bleeding or hematoma formation[a] | |
|   Wound (immediate or delayed) | 0.1–1 % |
| Further surgery (revision or hematoma drainage) | 0.1–1 % |
| *Less serious complications* | |
| Pain/discomfort/tenderness | |
|   Short term (<2 weeks) | 50–80 % |
| Cosmetic deformity | 0.1–1 % |

[a]Dependent on underlying pathology, anatomy, surgical technique, and preferences

**dysuria** is a consequence of surgery and is expected, but if prolonged beyond 72 h, it is abnormal. **Urinary tract infection** is very rare and may signify other underlying abnormalities, should it occur. **Bleeding** is rarely severe. **Recurrent meatal stenosis** is occasionally a problem that may require further surgical division.

---

**Consent and Risk Reduction**

**Main Points to Explain**

- GA risk
- Dysuria
- Pain/discomfort
- Bleeding/hematoma*
- Infection (urinary)
- Recurrent meatal stenosis
- Risks without surgery*

---

# Surgery for Hypospadias

## Description

General anesthesia is used. Hypospadias encompasses a range of congenital malformations of the position of the urethral opening on the ventral aspect of the penis. Hypospadias is usually identified at birth but may present with problems directing the stream of urine during micturition. The aim of surgery is to reposition the urethral opening closer to the tip of the penis and correct any chordee (curvature), and the associated dorsal hood of foreskin may be excised or used as skin flaps on the

**Table 7.3** Surgery for hypospadias estimated frequency of complications, risks, and consequences

| Complications, risks, and consequences | Estimated frequency |
|---|---|
| *Most significant/serious complications* | |
| Infection[a] overall | 1–5 % |
|   Subcutaneous | 1–5 % |
|   Urinary | 1–5 % |
| Significant bleeding or hematoma formation[a] | |
|   Wound (immediate or delayed) | 1–5 % |
| Wound breakdown/dehiscence | 1–5 % |
| Meatal ulceration/stenosis | 5–20 % |
| Urethral fistula | 5–20 % |
| Further surgery (other than urethral fistula)[a] | 1–5 % |
| *Less serious complications* | |
| Penile swelling | 50–80 % |
| Pain/discomfort/tenderness | |
|   Short term (<2 weeks) | >80 % |
| Urinary retention/catheterization | 0.1–1 % |
| Scarring/poor cosmesis (requiring revisional surgery) | 1–5 % |

[a]Dependent on underlying pathology, anatomy, surgical technique, and preferences

ventral aspect of the shaft of the penis after release of the chordee. The extent and type of surgery required depends on the type of hypospadias present, as does the range and severity of complications encountered after surgery. Glanular forms may require meatotomy alone with or without circumcision, whereas perineal or peno-scrotal forms may require extensive, multiple, staged surgical procedures. Transposition skin/mucosal flap repairs may be required. The relative risks and complications increase with the extent of surgery performed.

## Anatomical Points

Hypospadias is one of the most common congenital anomalies, occurring in about 1 in 300 male births. The anatomy can vary considerably, and the classification of hypospadias relates to the position of the urethral meatus. Four common types occur: glanular, penile, penoscrotal, and perineal, in descending order of frequency, with glanular and penile accounting for about 80 % of cases. The more severe the hypospadias, the more the downward curvature of the penis (chordee). In contrast, epispadias is where the urethral opening is on the dorsal surface of the penis and is very rare (sometimes associated with exstrophy of the bladder in severe forms).

## Perspective

See Table 7.3. Complications are generally minor; however, some may be more significant on occasions. These include infection, skin necrosis, cosmetic deformity, meatal ulceration, meatal stenosis, and bleeding. Urinary retention is not uncommon and occasionally requires catheterization (which may be done as part of some procedures to stent the urethra). Acute dysuria is a typical feature until the skin and mucosa heal. Bandaging in older boys should allow for expansion with erection, which can cause severe constrictive pain and require loosening and re-bandaging. Urethral fistula formation and meatal stenosis are the most common postoperative complications.

## Major Complications/Consequences

**Pain** may be significant and may require loosening of dressings and pain relief. **Acute dysuria** is a consequence of surgery and expected, but if prolonged beyond 5 days, it is abnormal. **Urinary tract infection** is rare. **Bleeding** is rarely severe. **Wound infection** usually responds to local dressings and oral antibiotics, if required. Infection may increase **scarring** and create **poor cosmesis**. **Meatal ulceration** may lead to **meatal stenosis** on occasions, which may require further surgery. **Urethral stenosis** can occur, depending on the degree of hypospadias, the surgery performed, and any infection. **Urethral fistula** can be a significant problem to deal with and may require repeated surgery. **Further revisional surgery** may be required, depending on the procedure performed and healing resulting in a poor cosmetic result.

**Consent and Risk Reduction**

**Main Points to Explain**

- GA risk
- Pain/discomfort
- Bleeding/hematoma*
- Meatal stenosis
- Infection (local/systemic)*
- Urethral fistula
- Penile scarring/deformity
- Urinary obstruction*
- Urine leakage*
- Possible further surgery*
- Risks without surgery*

## Surgery for Undescended Testes (Orchidopexy)

### Description

General anesthetic is used. The aim is to locate the testis that has partially descended or has failed to descend and attempt to mobilize the gonad into the scrotal sac, if this is achievable. In some cases, where this is not possible, orchidectomy is required, because of the increased risk of testicular carcinoma in an undescended testis. A transverse inguinal incision on the side of the undescended testis is usually used. The testis is usually surgically fixed in the scrotum by creating a dartos pouch. Laparoscopic approaches are progressively being used to locate an intra-abdominal testis as part of a first-stage procedure when high ligation of the testicular vessels is performed followed at a later date by an orchidopexy.

## Anatomical Points

The testis develops from the gonadal ridge, in a retroperitoneal position in the posterior abdominal wall, and usually descends caudally along the posterior abdominal wall across the ureter to reach the deep inguinal ring by about the 28th week of gestation. It carries with it its vascular and nerve supplies from the L1 and T10 levels, respectively. Migration of the testis then proceeds through the inguinal canal, collecting layers of spermatic fascia, and enters the scrotum at about the 32nd week. By full term, both testes are well down within the scrotum in 97 % of males and an even higher proportion by 3 months of age. True agenesis of the testis is very rare. The undescended testis usually lies in the upper scrotum or inguinal canal in the line of normal descent, in most cases. Ectopic testicular positioning occurs, with migration of the testis into the anterior abdominal, pubic, perineal, or thigh subcutaneous fatty tissues. The vascular supply to the testis is critical for the continued viability and function of the gonad.

## Perspective

See Table 7.4. Complications are generally minor; however, on occasions some may be more significant. These include bleeding, hematoma formation, infection, skin necrosis, wound dehiscence, acute and chronic pain, testicular ischemia, and atrophy. Infertility may be related to the initial maldescent, rather than the surgery. Urinary retention is rare and occasionally requires catheterization. The increased risk of testicular carcinoma is a consequence of the maldescent, not surgery.

## Major Complications/Consequences

**Pain** may be significant and may require support dressings and pain relief. **Bleeding** is rarely severe but can produce a large hematoma requiring surgical evacuation. **Testicular ischemia and atrophy** may occur and create **infertility** if the other testis is nonfunctional for any reason. **Testicular carcinoma** is a potential consequence

**Table 7.4** Surgery for undescended testes (orchidopexy) estimated frequency of complications, risks, and consequences

| Complications, risks, and consequences | Estimated frequency |
| --- | --- |
| *Most significant/serious complications* | |
| Infection[a] overall | 1–5 % |
|   Subcutaneous | 1–5 % |
|   Systemic sepsis[a] | <0.1 % |
| Scrotal swelling | 50–80 % |
| Testicular carcinoma (with failed orchidopexy or without surgery)[a] | 50–80 % |
| *Rare significant/serious problems* | |
| Bleeding or hematoma formation (scrotal, inguinal, or abdominal)[a] | |
|   Wound (immediate or delayed) | 0.1–1 % |
| Wound breakdown/dehiscence | 0.1–1 % |
| Wound sinus/suture granuloma | 0.1–1 % |
| Further surgery (revision or hematoma drainage) | 0.1–1 % |
| Testicular carcinoma (after successful orchidopexy)[a] | <0.1 % |
| *Less serious complications* | |
| Pain/discomfort/tenderness | |
|   Short term (<4 weeks) | 50–80 % |
|   Longer term (>12 weeks) | 0.1–1 % |
| Sensory changes | <0.1 % |
| Urinary retention/catheterization | 0.1–1 % |
| Scarring/poor cosmesis | <0.1 % |

[a]Dependent on underlying pathology, anatomy, surgical technique, and preferences

of a residual intra-abdominal testis, including the decision to defer or not operate. Even with orchidopexy, the rate of testicular carcinoma remains higher than for those with normal testicular descent. **Infection** usually responds to local dressings and oral antibiotics.

**Consent and Risk Reduction**

**Main Points to Explain**

- GA risk
- Pain/discomfort
- Bleeding/hematoma*
- Infection (local/urinary/systemic)*
- Infertility (possibility)
- Testicular cancer (possibility)
- Urinary obstruction*
- Possible further surgery*
- Risks without surgery*

# Circumcision

## Description

General anesthetic is usually used for adults and children, but when newborn infants are circumcised, a plastic ring device (Plastibell) local anesthetic cream or no anesthesia may be used. The aim is to remove the foreskin proximally to behind the glans penis. This exposes the glans permanently. Parental or religious preference is the usual indication in the newborn. Medical reasons for circumcision include severe phimosis (foreskin stenosis), recurrent urine infections or balanitis, balanitis xerotica obliterans (BXO), and paraphimosis where the foreskin is retracted and becomes stuck behind the glans. Acute paraphimosis can be treated with emergency initial reduction with sedation or a dorsal slit through the constricting band followed by a circumcision involving a GA.

## Anatomical Points

The foreskin ranges from minimal to very redundant, and physiological adhesions may join the glans penis to the foreskin in childhood which usually separate spontaneously before puberty. It is important to differentiate between the normal physiological phimosis of the young child and the pathological phimosis in older children which causes problems, such as balanitis.

## Perspective

See Table 7.5. Complications are generally minor and infrequent; however, some may be more significant on occasions. These include infection, cosmetic deformity, removing too much or too little skin, meatal ulceration, meatal stenosis, and bleeding. Urinary retention is uncommon and occasionally requires catheterization. Tight bandages especially with erections in the adolescent can be painful and require loosening and/or removal.

## Major Complications/Consequences

**Pain** may be significant and may require loosening of dressings and pain relief. **Bleeding** is rarely severe. **Infection** usually responds to local dressings and oral antibiotics, if required. Infection may increase **scarring** and create **poor**

**Table 7.5** Surgery for circumcision estimated frequency of complications, risks, and consequences

| Complications, risks, and consequences | Estimated frequency |
|---|---|
| *Most significant/serious complications* | |
| Infection[a] overall | 1–5 % |
|   Subcutaneous | 1–5 % |
|   Urinary | 1–5 % |
|   Systemic sepsis[a] | <0.1 % |
| Penile swelling | 50–80 % |
| *Rare significant/serious problems* | |
| Bleeding or hematoma formation[a] | |
|   Wound (immediate or delayed) | 0.1–1 % |
| Wound breakdown/dehiscence | 0.1–1 % |
| Meatal ulceration/stenosis | 0.1–1 % |
| Phimosis (constriction band formation covering the glans) | 0.1–1 % |
| Excessive removal of foreskin | 0.1–1 % |
| Further surgery (revision or hematoma drainage) | 0.1–1 % |
| *Less serious complications* | |
| Residual pain/discomfort/tenderness | |
|   Short term (<4 weeks) | 50–80 % |
|   Longer term (>12 weeks) | 0.1–1 % |
| Scarring/poor cosmesis | 0.1–1 % |

[a]Dependent on underlying pathology, anatomy, surgical technique, and preferences

**cosmesis**. **Meatal ulceration** may lead to **meatal stenosis** on occasions, which may require further surgery, e.g., meatotomy. **Cosmetic deformity** caused by **excess or too little shaft skin** or from **secondary phimosis** may occur and may require **revisional surgery**.

**Consent and Risk Reduction**

**Main Points to Explain**

- GA risk
- Pain/discomfort
- Ulceration (meatal/glans)
- Bleeding/hematoma*
- Infection (local/urinary/systemic)*
- Removing too much/too little skin
- Meatal stenosis
- Penile scarring/deformity
- Urinary obstruction*
- Possible further surgery*
- Risks without surgery*

## Bilateral Fixation of Testes/Exploration of the Testes (Testicular Torsion)

### Description

General anesthetic is used. The aim is to explore the scrotal contents, in particular the testes. The usual indication for bilateral fixation is proven or suspected torsion of one testis. Separate transverse scrotal incisions on each side or a single (transverse or midline) incision through the layers of the scrotum can be used to expose each testis and deliver it outside the scrotum for adequate inspection. The color of the testis is noted and any evidence of torsion. If the testis is black or dark, then a period of time is spent waiting for any color change and improvement in blood supply after reduction of the torsion. Most testes will regain a pink coloration; however, if established necrosis has occurred ($\sim > 6$ h ischemia time), then removal of the testis may be required. The objective is detorsion and fixation to prevent future torsion, achieved by several methods, which may fixate each testis to the scrotal median raphe or to the lateral scrotal tissues or both, or performing a Jaboulay procedure where the processus vaginalis is sutured behind the testis, thereby eradicating the space in which the testis can tort. Either nonabsorbable or absorbable sutures can be used.

### Anatomical Points

The main cause for testicular torsion is congenital high investment of the processus vaginalis around the spermatic cord and no attachment to the posterior epididymis, allowing the testis and epididymis to rotate. The anomaly often produces the clinical "bell clapper" testis phenomenon, with a classical "horizontal lie" of the testis. Focal tenderness over the upper epididymis may signify torsion of an appendage of the testis, but surgical exploration is typically warranted to confirm this. Doppler ultrasound is not very reliable in determining blood flow in children; it may be more helpful in the adolescent and mature male. Torsion of an undescended testis may occur in the younger child.

### Perspective

See Table 7.6. Complications are generally minor; however, on occasions some may be more significant. These include bleeding, hematoma formation, infection, acute short-term pain, and rarely recurrent torsion.

**Table 7.6** Surgery for testicular torsion estimated frequency of complications, risks, and consequences

| Complications, risks, and consequences | Estimated frequency |
|---|---|
| *Most significant/serious complications* | |
| Infection[a] overall | 1–5 % |
|    Subcutaneous | 1–5 % |
|    Systemic sepsis[a] | <0.1 % |
| Scrotal swelling | 50–80 % |
| Infertility/testicular atrophy[a] | 1–5 % |
| *Rare significant/serious problems* | |
| Bleeding or hematoma formation (scrotal)[a] | |
|    Wound (immediate or delayed) | 0.1–1 % |
| Wound breakdown/dehiscence | 0.1–1 % |
| Wound sinus/suture granuloma[a] | 0.1–1 % |
| Further surgery (revision or hematoma drainage) | 0.1–1 % |
| Recurrent torsion | <0.1 % |
| *Less serious complications* | |
| Pain/discomfort/tenderness | |
|    Short term (<4 weeks) | 50–80 % |
|    Longer term (>12 weeks) | 0.1–1 % |

[a]Dependent on underlying pathology, anatomy, surgical technique, and preferences

## *Major Complications/Consequences*

**Pain** may be significant and may require support dressings and pain relief. **Bleeding** is rarely severe but can produce a large hematoma requiring surgical evacuation. **Infection** usually responds to local dressings and oral antibiotics. **Infertility** may occur after surgery, if there has been bilateral torsion which is the reason the contralateral testis is fixed at the time of exploration for the torted testis.

### Consent and Risk Reduction

### Main Points to Explain

- GA risk
- Pain/discomfort
- Bleeding/hematoma*
- Infection (local/systemic)*
- Infertility (possibility)
- Urinary obstruction*
- Re-torsion (v. rare)
- Possible further surgery*
- Risks without surgery*

# Varicocele Repair: Open Inguinal

## Description

General anesthesia is used. The aim is to ligate the veins of the varicocele, to reduce the varicosities, and to lower the temperature around the testis. The main indications for surgery are to alleviate symptomatic pain and to encourage normal testicular development. Several techniques are used with the aim of ligation of the varicosities directly or the feeding veins more proximally. The ligation may be performed in the inguinal canal or retroperitoneum. Laparoscopic approaches for the latter are increasingly popular. Radiological embolization approaches are also used. For open surgery, an inguinal incision is made on the side of the pathology (>90 % left sided) approximately over the inguinal canal, and the external oblique fascia is opened. The procedure is usually unilateral, unless both sides are affected. If the varicocele is bilateral or right sided, it is important to exclude an intra-abdominal mass by performing an ultrasound of the abdomen.

## Anatomical Points

The testis is supplied principally by the testicular (aorta; L1) and cremasteric (inf. epigastric a.) arterial circulations, with a small contribution from the artery to the vas (from sup. vesical a.). The pampiniform plexus of draining testicular veins is the main source of varicosities constituting a varicocele. Ligation of the testicular vein in the inguinal region (before or in the inguinal canal) can reduce the varicosities, probably by reducing venous backflow due to gravity. Inadvertent injury or ligation of the adjacent testicular artery can produce testicular ischemia. Duplex ultrasound can be very reliable in determining anatomy and confirming the diagnosis. Varicoceles are more common on the left side due to a longer, more tortuous drainage route to the left renal vein. A simple varicocele usually collapses on lying down. Obstruction of the left testicular veins due to invasion of the left renal vein by a renal tumor may prevent the collapse of the varicocele on lying down.

## Perspective

See Table 7.7. Complications are generally minor; however, on occasions some may be more significant. These include bleeding, hematoma formation, infection, acute and chronic pain, and rarely ischemia of the testis. A potentially serious complication is infertility, due to ischemia of the testis after surgery; this may be significant if the other testis is also abnormal. Infertility may also result from the varicocele itself even though it is unilateral, possibly through temperature changes. Hydrocele is relatively common and may require further surgery.

**Table 7.7** Surgery for varicocele open repair estimated frequency of complications, risks, and consequences

| Complications, risks, and consequences | Estimated frequency |
| --- | --- |
| *Most significant/serious complications* | |
| Infection[a] overall | 1–5 % |
| Subcutaneous | 1–5 % |
| Systemic sepsis[a] | <0.1 % |
| Scrotal swelling[a] | 20–50 % |
| Hydrocele formation | 5–20 % |
| Recurrent varicocele[a] | 1–5 % |
| Further surgery (recurrent varicocele or hematoma drainage)[a] | 1–5 % |
| *Rare significant/serious problems* | |
| Bleeding or hematoma formation (scrotal, inguinal, or retroperitoneal)[a] | |
| Wound (immediate or delayed) | 0.1–1 % |
| Wound breakdown/dehiscence | 0.1–1 % |
| Testicular atrophy[a] | 0.1–1 % |
| Wound sinus/suture granuloma[a] | 0.1–1 % |
| Infertility[a] | <0.1 % |
| *Less serious complications* | |
| Pain/discomfort/tenderness | |
| Short term (<4 weeks) | 50–80 % |
| Longer term (>12 weeks) | 0.1–1 % |
| Urinary retention/catheterization | 0.1–1 % |
| Scarring/poor cosmesis | <0.1 % |

[a]Dependent on underlying pathology, anatomy, surgical technique, and preferences

## *Major Complications/Consequences*

**Pain** may be significant and may require support dressings and pain relief. **Chronic pain** occasionally occurs and is a major problem and may relate to testicular ischemia. **Bleeding** is rarely severe but can produce a **large hematoma** requiring surgical evacuation. **Infection** usually responds to local dressings and oral antibiotics. **Infertility** is a possible problem for men desiring childbearing ability. **Hydrocele formation** is not uncommon, perhaps due to lymphatic obstruction, and may require later surgery. **Recurrence of the varicocele** can occur.

---

**Consent and Risk Reduction**

**Main Points to Explain**

- GA risk
- Pain/discomfort
- Bleeding/hematoma*
- Infection (local/systemic)*
- Urinary obstruction*
- Hydrocele formation

- Recurrent varicocele
- Infertility (possibility)
- Possible further surgery*
- Risks without surgery*

## Varicocele Repair: Laparoscopic

### Description

General anesthesia is used. The aim is to ligate the testicular veins or testicular artery and vein to reduce the varicosities and lower the temperature of the ipsilateral testis. The main indications for surgery are to alleviate symptomatic pain and to encourage normal testicular development. Open approaches and radiological embolization approaches are also used. The ligation may be performed close to the inguinal canal or in the retroperitoneum. Surgery is performed on the side of the pathology (>90 % left sided), unless both sides are affected. If the varicocele is bilateral or right sided, it is important to exclude an intra-abdominal mass by performing an ultrasound of the abdomen.

### Anatomical Points

The testis is supplied principally by the testicular (aorta; L1) and cremasteric (inf. epigastric a.) arterial circulations, with a small contribution from the artery to the vas (from sup. vesical a.). The pampiniform plexus of draining testicular veins is the main source of varicosities constituting a varicocele. Ligation of the testicular vein in the inguinal region (before the inguinal canal) can reduce the varicosities, probably by reducing venous backflow due to gravity. Inadvertent injury or ligation of the testicular artery can produce testicular ischemia. Duplex ultrasound can be very reliable in determining anatomy and confirming the diagnosis. Varicoceles are more common on the left side due to a longer, more tortuous drainage route to the left renal vein. A simple varicocele usually collapses on lying down. Obstruction of the left testicular veins due to invasion of the left renal vein by renal tumor may prevent the collapse of the varicocele on lying down.

### Perspective

See Table 7.8. Complications are generally minor; however, on occasions some may be more significant. These include bleeding, hematoma formation, infection, acute and chronic pain, and rarely ischemia of the testis. A potentially serious complication is infertility, due to ischemia of the testis after surgery; this may be significant

**Table 7.8**  Surgery for varicocele laparoscopic repair estimated frequency of complications, risks, and consequences

| Complications, risks, and consequences | Estimated frequency |
|---|---|
| ***Most significant/serious complications*** | |
| Infection[a] overall | 1–5 % |
|    Subcutaneous | 1–5 % |
|    Systemic sepsis[a] | <0.1 % |
| Scrotal swelling[a] | 50–80 % |
| Scrotal and subcutaneous emphysema[a] | 5–20 % |
| Hydrocele formation | 5–20 % |
| Recurrent varicocele[a] | 1–5 % |
| Further surgery (recurrent varicocele or hematoma drainage)[a] | 1–5 % |
| ***Rare significant/serious problems*** | |
| Bleeding or hematoma formation (scrotal, inguinal, or retroperitoneal)[a] | |
|    Wound, port sites (immediate or delayed) | 0.1–1 % |
| Major vascular or bowel injury | 0.1–1 % |
| Wound breakdown/dehiscence | 0.1–1 % |
| Seroma formation[a] | 0.1–1 % |
| Testicular atrophy[a] | 0.1–1 % |
| Wound sinus/suture granuloma[a] | 0.1–1 % |
| Gas embolism | <0.1 % |
| Infertility[a] | <0.1 % |
| ***Less serious complications*** | |
| Pain/discomfort/tenderness | |
|    Short term (<4 weeks) | 50–80 % |
|    Longer term (>12 weeks) | 0.1 % |
| Urinary retention/catheterization | 0.1–1 % |
| Scarring/poor cosmesis | <0.1 % |

[a]Dependent on underlying pathology, anatomy, surgical technique, and preferences

if the other testis is abnormal. Complications from insertion of the ports and instruments, and gas insufflation, can occur but are rare. Gas embolism is exceedingly rare but potentially catastrophic, while subcutaneous gas emphysema is more common and usually resolves spontaneously. Hydrocele is relatively common and may require further surgery.

## *Major Complications/Consequences*

**Pain** may be significant and may require support dressings and pain relief. **Chronic pain** occasionally occurs and may relate to testicular ischemia. **Bleeding** is rarely severe but can produce a **large hematoma** requiring surgical evacuation. **Infection** usually responds to local dressings and oral antibiotics. **Infertility** is a possible problem for men desiring childbearing ability, possibly through temperature changes. **Hydrocele formation** is not uncommon, perhaps due to lymphatic obstruction, and may require surgery. **Recurrence of the varicocele** can occur.

**Consent and Risk Reduction**

**Main Points to Explain**

- GA risk
- Pain/discomfort
- Bleeding/hematoma*
- Infection (local/systemic)*
- Urinary obstruction*
- Hydrocele formation
- Recurrent varicocele
- Infertility (possibility) gas embolism
- Groin scarring/deformity
- Possible further surgery*
- Risks without surgery*

# Surgery for Posterior Urethral Valves

## Description

General anesthetic is usually used. Obstruction of the posterior urethra due to congenital "valves" is the most common cause of bladder outflow obstruction in the newborn male and is often detected on antenatal ultrasound screening. Severe obstruction to bladder outflow can produce dilatation of the ureters and renal pelves due to either vesicoureteric reflux or vesicoureteric junction obstruction which may result in the development of renal failure. The aim of surgery is to identify the cause of the urethral obstruction with cystoscopy, and if posterior urethral valves are confirmed and depending on the size of the infant, the valve leaflets are endoscopically incised via the cystoscope using diathermy. Inadequate resection may occur especially in the small infant when visibility may be poor. Temporary diversion is then often performed by creating a vesicostomy, where the bladder is opened onto the lower abdominal wall, thereby bypassing the urethra until renal function is stabilized and the child has grown. Severe obstruction may occur in utero and if untreated can be lethal before or shortly after birth. Early in utero surgery has been performed in selected cases but may not improve overall clinical outcome.

## Anatomical Points

The bladder and urethra develop from the urogenital sinus by about the 12th week of gestation. Some of the urethral lining tissue may form valve-like structures, known as posterior urethral valves, causing urethral outflow obstruction. The exact embryology of the development of the posterior urethral valve leaflets is unknown.

**Table 7.9** Surgery for posterior urethral valves estimated frequency of complications, risks, and consequences

| Complications, risks, and consequences | Estimated frequency |
|---|---|
| *Most significant/serious complications* | |
| Infection[a] overall | 1–5 % |
|    Systemic sepsis secondary to a urine infection | 1–5 % |
| Damage to external sphincter | 1–5 % |
| Progressive renal failure[a] | 1–5 % |
| *Rare significant/serious problems* | |
| Recurrent obstruction[a] | 0.1–1 % |
| Urethral or bladder perforation[a] | 0.1–1 % |
| Further surgery (revision)[a] | 0.1–1 % |
| *Less serious complications* | |
| Pain/discomfort/tenderness | |
|    Short term (<4 weeks) | 20–50 % |
|    Longer term (>12 weeks) | 0.1–1 % |
| Urinary retention/catheterization | >80 % |

[a]Dependent on underlying pathology, anatomy, surgical technique, and preferences

## Perspective

See Table 7.9. Complications are generally minor; however, on occasions some may be more significant. These include bleeding and infection. Urinary catheterization is often performed, as without catheterization urinary retention is not uncommon from edema at the site of valve resection. Progressive renal failure can occur but relates to the degree of renal dysplasia that occurred prior to birth and in the long-term to the poorly compliant high-pressure "valve bladder," rather than the actual surgery.

## Major Complications

Rarely, **urethral perforation** and **bladder injury** may occur and are perhaps the most significant complications. **Infection** may ensue usually responding to antibiotics. Infection may cause further damage to the kidneys rarely scarring at the site of valve resection. **Bleeding** is rarely severe. **Renal failure** may not always be reversed by surgery and may relate to the renal dysplasia. **Pain** is not usually severe in the newborn.

---

**Consent and Risk Reduction**

**Main Points to Explain**

- GA risk
- Pain/discomfort
- Bleeding/hematoma*
- Infection (local/systemic)*
- Recurrent urinary obstruction*

- Urine leakage*
- Urine collection*
- Urethral stenosis
- Urethral perforation
- Bladder injury
- Risk of other abdominal organ injury*
- Progressive renal failure (possibility)
- Possible further surgery*
- Risks without surgery*

## Surgery for Ureteric Reimplantation

### Description

General anesthetic is usually used. Vesicoureteric reflux (VUR) is the most common underlying congenital anomaly in children who present with urinary tract infections. Reflux nephropathy is a major consequence of moderate to severe vesicoureteric reflux and repeated urinary tract infections. Other renal tract anomalies may be associated. Severe reflux can produce dilatation of the ureters and renal pelves with clubbing of the calyces and thinning of the renal parenchyma. Eighty percent of VUR is mild to moderate, and in 80 % of these children, the VUR will spontaneously resolve. Antibiotic treatment may be used in mild to moderate grades of VUR, but surgical intervention is often required in the severe grades of VUR particularly when there is an associated structural abnormality. The aim of surgery is to reimplant the ureter(s) to recreate the valve-like function by creating a submucosal tunnel across the bladder base and thereby eliminate vesicoureteric reflux. Laparoscopic methods have been used but are not yet proven to be reliable. Endoscopic injection of "Deflux" under the refluxing ureteric orifice is used in specific cases, but as yet long-term follow-up is not available.

### Anatomical Points

The bladder develops from the urogenital sinus by about the 12th week of gestation, and the ureter forms from the mesonephric duct and enters the developing kidney which lies adjacent to the bladder. The ureter usually enters the bladder wall at an angle, surrounded by the bladder smooth muscle and then entering the bladder through a submucosal tunnel, which creates a valve to prevent urine flowing retrogradely as the bladder fills and contracts to empty.

**Table 7.10** Surgery for ureteric reimplantation estimated frequency of complications, risks, and consequences

| Complications, risks, and consequences | Estimated frequency |
|---|---|
| *Most significant/serious complications* | |
| Infection[a] overall | 1–5 % |
|   Subcutaneous | 1–5 % |
|   Abscess formation | 0.1–1 % |
|   Systemic sepsis[a] | <0.1 % |
| Ureteric obstruction[a] | 1–5 % |
| *Rare significant/serious problems* | |
| Bleeding and hematoma formation (bladder, peritoneal, pre-peritoneal)[a] | |
|   Wound (immediate or delayed) | 0.1–1 % |
| Urine leakage | 0.1–1 % |
| Urine collection (urinoma) | 0.1–1 % |
| Ureteric perforation[a] | 0.1–1 % |
| Bladder perforation[a] | 0.1–1 % |
| Recurrent reflux | 0.1–1 % |
| Further surgery (revision of ureteric reimplantation) | 0.1–1 % |
| *Less serious complications* | |
| Pain/discomfort/tenderness | |
|   Short term (<4 weeks) | 20–50 % |
|   Longer term (>12 weeks) | 0.1–1 % |
| Urinary retention/catheterization | 0.1–1 % |

[a]Dependent on underlying pathology, anatomy, surgical technique, and preferences

## Perspective

See Table 7.10. Complications are generally minor; however, on occasions some may be more significant. These include bleeding, hematoma formation, urine and wound infection, abscess formation, and acute and chronic pain. Urinary catheterization is usually performed at the time of surgery when closing the bladder. Occasionally, placement of a ureteric stent past the anastomosis at the reimplanted VUJ may be done to ensure adequate drainage particularly if there is a single kidney or neurogenic bladder. Without catheterization, urinary retention secondary to clots may occur. Dysuria is not uncommon and bladder spasms causing bladder pain may occur.

## Major Complications/Consequences

**Urine leakage** and **urine collection (urinoma) formation** may occur and is perhaps the most significant complication. **Drainage** of the collection may be required, especially if secondarily infected. **Infection** may ensue, usually responding to antibiotics, but **abscess formation** rarely occurs. Infection may cause

**scarring** and create **recurrent VUJ stenosis** resulting in urine infections. **Bleeding** is rarely severe but can produce a hematoma, requiring surgical evacuation, which may become secondarily infected. **Renal failure due to reflux-associated nephropathy**, if established, may not be reversed by the surgery. **Pain** may be significant and require regular pain relief. **Chronic pain** is rarely a major problem. **Further surgery** may be needed for **recurrent vesicoureteric reflux** or vesicoureteric junction obstruction.

---

**Consent and Risk Reduction**

**Main Points to Explain**

- GA risk
- Pain/discomfort
- Bleeding/hematoma*
- Infection (local/systemic)*
- Urinary obstruction*
- Urine leakage and collection*
- Recurrent urinary obstruction
- Risk of other abdominal organ injury*
- Possible further surgery*
- Risks without surgery*

---

# Pyeloplasty Surgery

## *Description*

General anesthetic is used. Pelviureteric obstruction is caused by narrowing of the pelviureteric junction (PUJ). The obstruction may be intrinsic, intramural, or extrinsic. Intrinsic causes may be a calculus, extrinsic due to an anomalous vessel crossing the ureter, or the most common is intramural, where there is a narrowed segment of ureter at the PUJ. Recurrent renal infection may occur, particularly when there is associated vesicoureteric reflux (VUR; 25–30 % cases). Severe obstruction will produce dilatation of the renal pelvis extending into the calyces, thinning the renal parenchyma with eventual deterioration in renal function. The aim of surgery is to identify the site(s) of obstruction, remove the narrowed segment at the PUJ, and reanastomose the ureter to the renal pelvis – a pyeloplasty. Laparoscopic pyeloplasty is performed in some centers, particularly in the older age group, with equivalent functional success as compared to an open pyeloplasty. Transureteric endoscopic surgical approaches have been performed but without good long-term success rates; they are no longer recommended.

**Table 7.11** Surgery for pyeloplasty estimated frequency of complications, risks, and consequences

| Complications, risks, and consequences | Estimated frequency |
|---|---|
| *Most significant/serious complications* | |
| Infection[a] overall | 1–5 % |
| Subcutaneous | 1–5 % |
| Urinary | 1–5 % |
| Abscess formation | <0.1 % |
| Systemic sepsis[a] | <0.1 % |
| Bleeding and hematoma formation (renal pelvicalyceal, retro-/intraperitoneal)[a] | |
| Wound (immediate or delayed) | 1–5 % |
| *Rare significant/serious problems* | |
| Urine leakage[a] | 0.1–1 % |
| Urine collection (urinoma)[a] | 0.1–1 % |
| Recurrent obstruction[a] | 0.1–1 % |
| Further surgery (revision or hematoma drainage)[a] | 0.1–1 % |
| *Less serious complications* | |
| Pain/discomfort/tenderness | |
| Short term (<4 weeks) | 20–50 % |
| Longer term (>12 weeks) | 0.1–1 % |
| Sensory changes associated with the wound | <0.1 % |
| Urinary retention/catheterization | <0.1 % |

[a]Dependent on underlying pathology, anatomy, surgical technique, and preferences

## *Anatomical Points*

The kidneys develop in three successive stages between the 4th and 8th week of gestation: pronephros, mesonephros, and metanephros. After the ureter has entered the kidney, it will then migrate to about the L1–L2 level by birth lying on the posterior abdominal wall. The blood supply to the kidney and ureter changes as the kidney ascends from the pelvis to the L1–L2 level, and often there may be a second renal vessel supplying the lower pole of the kidney, which may cause compression at the pelviureteric junction if it crosses the ureter. Horseshoe kidneys and the lower pole of a duplex kidney are particularly associated with PUJ obstructions caused by aberrant blood vessels.

Hydronephrosis secondary to a PUJ obstruction may be diagnosed on antenatal ultrasound. Investigations performed to confirm the diagnosis are an ultrasound, Mag3renal nuclide scan, and occasionally microscopy and culture of urine (MCU) if there are suspicions of associated VUR.

## *Perspective*

See Table 7.11. Complications are generally minor. Urine leakage and formation of a urine collection (urinoma) can occur. This may become secondarily infected. Placement of a ureteric stent across the anastomosis of the reconstructed PUJ with or without a urethral catheter may be used during surgery, dependent on surgeon preference, to ensure adequate drainage.

## Major Complications

Rarely, **urine leakage** and **urine collection (urinoma) formation** may occur and is perhaps the most significant complication as it may result in the development of a secondary PUJ obstruction which requires revision surgery. **Bleeding** is rarely severe. **Renal injury** or **injury to other abdominal organs is rare. Further surgery** may be needed for **recurrent PUJ obstruction**.

---

**Consent and Risk Reduction**

**Main Points to Explain**

- GA risk
- Pain/discomfort
- Bleeding/hematoma*
- Infection (local/systemic)*
- Recurrent urinary obstruction*
- Urine leakage and collection*
- Risk of renal or other abdominal organ injury*
- Possible blood transfusion
- Possible tumor recurrence*
- Possible further surgery*
- Risks without surgery*

---

# Nephrectomy or Partial Nephrectomy: Open or Laparoscopic

## Description

General anesthesia is used. The usual indications for a *nephrectomy* are a poorly functioning, congenitally abnormal kidney, e.g., multicystic dysplastic kidney, PUJ obstruction, and Wilms' tumor. Other indications are end-stage kidney disease with renal hypertension, a nonfunctioning atrophic kidney secondary to VUR, an obstructed kidney with recurrent infections, cystic kidney disease with symptoms, or a living related transplant donor nephrectomy. Indications for *partial nephrectomy* are small renal tumors or nonfunctioning segments of duplex kidneys. The aim of the procedure is to remove the affected kidney (totally or partially). Complete removal of the ureter is only necessary with distended ureters in duplex kidneys or in association with VUR.

Partial nephrectomy and complete nephrectomy for congenital and/or benign disease are performed via a posterolateral, retroperitoneal approach.

When removing a malignant Wilms' tumor, an open anterior transperitoneal approach is used to allow staging of the tumor with a formal laparotomy and excision of lymph nodes along the aorta. Wilms' tumor is usually very sensitive to chemotherapy, so if the tumor is very large at presentation or if there is extension into the renal vein or IVC, then preoperative chemotherapy after tumor biopsy would be indicated.

Laparoscopic nephrectomy or partial nephrectomy is a very appropriate option for the removal of congenitally abnormal kidneys, which are usually atrophic and small. The laparoscopic approach is usually retroperitoneal, but if access to the pelvis is required to completely remove the ureter, then a transperitoneal approach would be used. There are no significant postoperative issues when comparing laparoscopic and open nephrectomy for benign renal lesions. Laparoscopic nephrectomy for Wilms' tumors is contraindicated.

## Anatomical Points

**See Note in pyeloplasty.** The kidneys develop in three successive stages between the 4th and 8th week of gestation: pronephros, mesonephros, and metanephros. After the ureter has entered the kidney, it will then migrate to about the L1–L2 level by birth lying on the posterior abdominal wall. The blood supply to the kidney and ureter changes as the kidney ascends from the pelvis to the L1–L2 level, and often there may be a second renal vessel supplying the lower pole of the kidney, which may cause compression at the pelviureteric junction if it crosses the ureter. Horseshoe kidneys and the lower pole of a duplex kidney are particularly associated with PUJ obstructions caused by aberrant blood vessels.

Hydronephrosis secondary to a PUJ obstruction may be diagnosed on antenatal ultrasound. Investigations performed to confirm the diagnosis are an ultrasound, Mag3renal nuclide scan, and occasionally microscopy and culture of urine (MCU) if there are suspicions of associated VUR. For a renal tumor, the anatomical extent and the displacement or involvement of adjacent organs largely determines the surgery required, and this may be reasonably planned preoperatively using ultrasound and CT or MRI.

## Perspective

See Table 7.12. Significant bleeding and injury to adjacent structures are rare. Small bowel obstruction due to postoperative adhesions is very uncommon but can occur after transperitoneal surgery. Retroperitoneal surgery for small poorly functioning kidneys in children is usually well tolerated with minimal side effects. This usually requires an overnight stay in hospital, and normal longer-term survival with a single

**Table 7.12** Surgery for open and laparoscopic nephrectomy or partial nephrectomy estimated frequency of complications, risks, and consequences

| Complications, risks, and consequences | Estimated frequency |
|---|---|
| *Most significant/serious complications* | |
| Infection[a] | |
|    Subcutaneous/wound | 1–5 % |
|    Urinary/systemic | 1–5 % |
|    Chest infection | 1–5 % |
|    Basal atelectasis | 5–20 % |
| Bleeding/hematoma[a] | 1–5 % |
| Paralytic ileus[b] | |
|    With flank approach | 0.1–1 % |
|    With transabdominal approach | 1–5 % |
| Urine leakage/collection (urinoma)[a] | 1–5 % |
| Small bowel obstruction (early or late)[a] | <0.1 % |
| *Rare significant/serious problems* | |
| Bowel injury (stomach, duodenum, small bowel, colon)[b] | <0.1 % |
| *Less serious complications* | |
| Pain/discomfort/tenderness | |
|    Short term (<4 weeks) | 20–50 % |
|    Longer term (>12 weeks) | 0.1–1 % |
| Urinary retention/catheterization | 0.1–1 % |
| Wound scarring (deformity/dimpling of wound scar/poor cosmesis) | <1 % |
| *Laparoscopic specific complications* | |
| Conversion to open operation | 1–5 % |
| Injury to the bowel or blood vessels (trocar or diathermy) | 0.1–1 % |
|    Duodenal/gastric/small bowel/colonic/iliac/mesenteric | |
| Gas embolus | 0.1–1 % |
| Pneumothorax | 0.1–1 % |
| Deep venous thrombosis/pulmonary embolism | 0.1–1 % |

[a]Dependent on underlying pathology, surgical technique preferences
[b]Incision used, and location on the body

kidney is typical. There are usually no lifestyle restrictions recommended with a single normal kidney, perhaps barring involvement in vigorous contact sport at an elite level, e.g., the Olympics. Larger, open operations usually have increased associated risks, often depending on the operative indication. With any laparoscopic surgery, the patient should be prewarned of the risk of conversion to an open procedure.

## Major Complications/Consequences

**Bleeding** is one of the major potential complications of nephrectomy. **Transfusion** is rarely required for nephrectomy and blood would not normally be grouped and matched unless it was a large malignant tumor. Late mortality from Wilms' tumor is due to **tumor spread. Small bowel obstruction** may be a recurrent issue after transperitoneal nephrectomy, often treated conservatively, but surgery may be required to separate the adhesions. Infection may occasionally lead to **systemic sepsis** and even **multisystem organ failure** is rare but is a significant cause of early **mortality** when it occurs. Later mortality is due to **tumor recurrence or persistence**. **Pancreatic leak**, collection, and **fistula** are very rare. **Specific complications of partial nephrectomy** are urinary bleeding (**macroscopic hematuria**) and/or **urine extravasation**. Both may successfully be treated conservatively or may require endoscopic ureteric stenting, endovascular embolization, or open revision. **Peritonitis** can also be a significant complication. For <u>laparoscopic approaches</u>, **port site hernia formation** can occur. **Gas embolism, major vascular injury**, and **bowel injury** are very rare. **Bowel injury** may very rarely require **stoma formation**. Wilms' tumor in children is responsive to chemotherapy, and dependent on the stage of the tumor, radiotherapy may also be required, in addition to surgery and chemotherapy.

---

**Consent and Risk Reduction**

**Main Points to Explain**

- GA risk
- Pain/discomfort
- Bleeding/hematoma*
- Infection (local/systemic)*
- Urinary obstruction*
- Urine leakage and collection*
- Risk of other abdominal organ injury*
- Respiratory complications
- Small bowel obstruction (open surgery)*
- Possible tumor recurrence*
- Renal failure (possible, late)
- Possible blood transfusion
- Possible further surgery*
- Risks without surgery*

**\*Dependent on pathology and type of surgery performed**

---

# Further Reading, References, and Resources

## *Surgery for Labial Fusion/Adhesions*

Acer T, Otgün I, Oztürk O, Kocabaş T, Tezcan AY, Cirak A, Oney MD, Kantar B, Hiçsönmez A. Do hygienic factors affect labial fusion recurrence? A search for possible related etiologic factors. J Pediatr Surg. 2012;47(10):1913–8.

Coran AG, Adzick NS, Krummel TM, Laberge J-M, Shamberger R, Caldamone A. Pediatric surgery, 2-volume set: expert consult – online and print. 7th ed. Philadelphia: Elsevier; 2012.

Gearhart JG, Rink RC, Mouriquand PDE. Pediatric urology. 2nd ed. Philadelphia: Saunders; 2009. ISBN 9781416032045.

Mayoglou L, Dulabon L, Martin-Alguacil N, Pfaff D, Schober J. Success of treatment modalities for labial fusion: a retrospective evaluation of topical and surgical treatments. J Pediatr Adolesc Gynecol. 2009;22(4):247–50.

Spitz L, Coran AG. Operative pediatric surgery. 7th ed. Boca Raton: CRC Press; 2013.

## Surgery for Meatal Stenosis

Coran AG, Adzick NS, Krummel TM, Laberge J-M, Shamberger R, Caldamone A. Pediatric surgery, 2-volume set: expert consult – online and print. 7th ed. Philadelphia: Elsevier; 2012.

Gearhart JG, Rink RC, Mouriquand PDE. Pediatric urology. 2nd ed. Philadelphia: Saunders; 2009. ISBN 9781416032045.

Singh RB, Pavithran NM. Lessons learnt from Snodgrass tip urethroplasty: a study of 75 cases. Pediatr Surg Int. 2004;20(3):204–6.

Spitz L, Coran AG. Operative pediatric surgery. 7th ed. Boca Raton: CRC Press; 2013.

## Surgery for Hypospadias

Arnaud A, Harper L, Aulagne MB, Michel JL, Maurel A, Dobremez E, Fourcade L, Andriamananarivo L. Choosing a technique for severe hypospadias. Afr J Paediatr Surg. 2011; 8(3):286–90.

Bracka A. A versatile two-stage hypospadias repair. Br J Plast Surg. 1995;48:345–52.

Castagnetti M, El Ghoneimi A. Surgical management of primary severe hypospadias in children: systematic 20-year review. J Urol. 2010;184:1469–75.

Coran AG, Adzick NS, Krummel TM, Laberge J-M, Shamberger R, Caldamone A. Pediatric surgery, 2-volume set: expert consult – online and print. 7th ed. Philadelphia: Elsevier; 2012.

Dewan PA, Dinneen MD, Winkle D, Duffy PG, Ransley PG. Hypospadias: Duckett pedicle tube urethroplasty. Eur Urol. 1991;20:39–42.

Duckett Jr JW. Transverse preputial island flap technique for repair of severe hypospadias. J Urol. 1995;153:1660–3.

Gearhart JG, Rink RC, Mouriquand PDE. Pediatric urology. 2nd ed. Philadelphia: Saunders; 2009. ISBN 9781416032045.

Gorduza DB, Gay CL, de Mattos ES, Demede D, Hameury F, Berthiller J, et al. Does androgen stimulation prior to hypospadias surgery increase the rate of healing complications? – A preliminary report. J Pediatr Urol. 2011;7:158–61.

Spitz L, Coran AG. Operative pediatric surgery. 7th ed. Boca Raton: CRC Press; 2013.

Wilkinson DJ, Farrelly P, Kenny SE. Outcomes in distal hypospadias: a systematic review of the Mathieu and tubularized incised plate repairs. J Pediatr Urol. 2012;8(3):307–12.

## Surgery for Undescended Testes (Orchidopexy)

Coran AG, Adzick NS, Krummel TM, Laberge J-M, Shamberger R, Caldamone A. Pediatric surgery, 2-volume set: expert consult – online and print. 7th ed. Philadelphia: Elsevier; 2012.

Gearhart JG, Rink RC, Mouriquand PDE. Pediatric urology. 2nd ed. Philadelphia: Saunders; 2009. ISBN 9781416032045.

Spitz L, Coran AG. Operative pediatric surgery. 7th ed. Boca Raton: CRC Press; 2013.

## *Surgery for Circumcision*

Coran AG, Adzick NS, Krummel TM, Laberge J-M, Shamberger R, Caldamone A. Pediatric surgery, 2-volume set: expert consult – online and print. 7th ed. Philadelphia: Elsevier; 2012.
Gearhart JG, Rink RC, Mouriquand PDE. Pediatric urology. 2nd ed. Philadelphia: Saunders; 2009. ISBN 9781416032045.
Spitz L, Coran AG. Operative pediatric surgery. 7th ed. Boca Raton: CRC Press; 2013.

## *Bilateral Fixation of Testes/Exploration of Testes (Testicular Torsion)*

Coran AG, Adzick NS, Krummel TM, Laberge J-M, Shamberger R, Caldamone A. Pediatric surgery, 2-volume set: expert consult – online and print. 7th ed. Philadelphia: Elsevier; 2012.
Gearhart JG, Rink RC, Mouriquand PDE. Pediatric urology. 2nd ed. Philadelphia: Saunders; 2009. ISBN 9781416032045.
Spitz L, Coran AG. Operative pediatric surgery. 7th ed. Boca Raton: CRC Press; 2013.

## *Varicocele Repair: Open Inguinal*

Coran AG, Adzick NS, Krummel TM, Laberge J-M, Shamberger R, Caldamone A. Pediatric surgery, 2-volume set: expert consult – online and print. 7th ed. Philadelphia: Elsevier; 2012.
Gearhart JG, Rink RC, Mouriquand PDE. Pediatric urology. 2nd ed. Philadelphia: Saunders; 2009. ISBN 9781416032045.
Spitz L, Coran AG. Operative pediatric surgery. 7th ed. Boca Raton: CRC Press; 2013.

## *Varicocele Repair: Laparoscopic*

Coran AG, Adzick NS, Krummel TM, Laberge J-M, Shamberger R, Caldamone A. Pediatric surgery, 2-volume set: expert consult – online and print. 7th ed. Philadelphia: Elsevier; 2012.
Gearhart JG, Rink RC, Mouriquand PDE. Pediatric urology. 2nd ed. Philadelphia: Saunders; 2009. ISBN 9781416032045.
Spitz L, Coran AG. Operative pediatric surgery. 7th ed. Boca Raton: CRC Press; 2013.

## *Surgery for Posterior Urethral Valves*

Coran AG, Adzick NS, Krummel TM, Laberge J-M, Shamberger R, Caldamone A. Pediatric surgery, 2-volume set: expert consult – online and print. 7th ed. Philadelphia: Elsevier; 2012.
Churchill BM, Krueger RP, Fleisher MH, Hardy BE. Complications of posterior urethral valve surgery and their prevention. Urol Clin North Am. 1983;10(3):519–30.
Gearhart JG, Rink RC, Mouriquand PDE. Pediatric urology. 2nd ed. Philadelphia: Saunders; 2009. ISBN 9781416032045.

Lopez Pereira P, Martinez Urrutia MJ, Jaureguizar E. Initial and long-term management of posterior urethral valves. World J Urol. 2004;22(6):418–24. Review.

Schober JM, Dulabon LM, Woodhouse CR. Outcome of valve ablation in late-presenting posterior urethral valves. BJU Int. 2004;94(4):616–9.

Spitz L, Coran AG. Operative pediatric surgery. 7th ed. Boca Raton: CRC Press; 2013.

Warren J, Pike JG, Leonard MP. Posterior urethral valves in Eastern Ontario – a 30 year perspective. Can J Urol. 2004;11(2):2210–5.

## Surgery for Ureteric Reimplantation

Coran AG, Adzick NS, Krummel TM, Laberge J-M, Shamberger R, Caldamone A. Pediatric surgery, 2-volume set: expert consult – online and print. 7th ed. Philadelphia: Elsevier; 2012.

Gearhart JG, Rink RC, Mouriquand PDE. Pediatric urology. 2nd ed. Philadelphia: Saunders; 2009. ISBN 9781416032045.

Spitz L, Coran AG. Operative pediatric surgery. 7th ed. Boca Raton: CRC Press; 2013.

## Surgery for Pyeloplasty

Coran AG, Adzick NS, Krummel TM, Laberge J-M, Shamberger R, Caldamone A. Pediatric surgery, 2-volume set: expert consult – online and print. 7th ed. Philadelphia: Elsevier; 2012.

Gearhart JG, Rink RC, Mouriquand PDE. Pediatric urology. 2nd ed. Philadelphia: Saunders; 2009. ISBN 9781416032045.

Spitz L, Coran AG. Operative pediatric surgery. 7th ed. Boca Raton: CRC Press; 2013.

## Nephrectomy and Partial Nephrectomy: Open and Laparoscopic

Coran AG, Adzick NS, Krummel TM, Laberge J-M, Shamberger R, Caldamone A. Pediatric surgery, 2-volume set: expert consult – online and print. 7th ed. Philadelphia: Elsevier; 2012.

Gearhart JG, Rink RC, Mouriquand PDE. Pediatric urology. 2nd ed. Philadelphia: Saunders; 2009. ISBN 9781416032045.

Spitz L, Coran AG. Operative pediatric surgery. 7th ed. Boca Raton: CRC Press; 2013.

# Index

Printed in the United States
By Bookmasters